# THIN
*In 30 Minutes*

# THIN
## In 30 Minutes

**Walk Your Way THIN
in Just 30 Minutes or Less**

**Job Benson and Andrea Albright**

All rights reserved. No part of this book or lifestyle system may be reproduced or transmitted in any manner or form whatsoever without written permission, except in the case of brief quotations used in books, articles or newspapers.

This walking protocol is intended as a reference guide for daily exercise. It is not a medical manual to replace the advice of your physician or to substitute any treatment prescribed by your physician. If you are diagnosed as ill or feel that you may have any undiagnosed medical problem, we emphatically urge you to consult with your medical, health or other competent professional before adopting any of the suggestions in *Walk Your Way Thin* or drawing any inferences from the information we are offering.

If you are taking prescription medications, you should never change your diet (making it better or worse) without consulting with your physician, because dietary fluctuations can affect the metabolism of the drugs you are taking. This book, system and the author's opinion are solely for informational and educational purposes. I am not intending to diagnose or treat any medical conditions. The author disclaims all responsibility for any liability, loss or risk, personal or otherwise, which might be incurred as a consequence, directly or indirectly, of the use and application of any of the contents of this book or system.

The author does not directly or indirectly prescribe or dispense medical advice or prescribe the use of diet, exercise or supplements without medical approval. Doctors, nutritionists and other experts in the field of diet, health and nutrition hold widely varying views. The author's intent is only to offer health information and research to help you cooperate with your medical or health advisors in your mutual quest to improve your health. In the event that you use this information without your doctors' approval, you are prescribing for yourself. This is your Constitutional right, and the author assumes no responsibility.

FITOLOGY LLC.
4100 West Eldorado Parkway
Suite 100-401
McKinney, TX 75070


Copyright © 2012 Fitology/Velocity House
ALL RIGHTS RESERVED

ISBN: 978-1-62409-004-2

# A Personal Introduction from the Author

Walking for greater weight loss and more energy seems almost too good to be true, and I had my doubts until my husband showed me how it was done and the science behind it. Now I'm seeing proof that you don't have to work hard to get great results.

I've struggled with my weight since I was a teenager, and coming from an obese family background, I was determined to not let it happen to me. After years of yo-yo dieting, I finally discovered the secrets to natural weight loss, and I went from a size 12 to a healthy size 2, but I had to really "work" for it. I spent hours doing intense cardio and running, because I thought that the harder I pushed, the more fat I would burn off. Geez, that was exhausting!

No matter how hard I ran, if I stopped for a few days or went on vacation, I would gain it all back (so depressing!). No matter what I did, I still had stubborn "pockets" of body fat on my upper thighs, inner thighs, arms and that below-the-belly-button belly pooch that wouldn't go away, no matter how many sit-ups and hours of intense exercise I did.

Then I met my husband, and I started following his advice about walking for fat burning, and those stubborn pockets of body fat are disappearing! Even better, I'm spending less time and energy on the treadmill than ever before.

I am an avid believer in walking to get better weight loss, and I'll never go back to those old days of exhausting myself on a treadmill again. I'm 34 years young, and feel fitter, leaner and healthier than I did in my 20s. You can do this at any age!

One of my favorite things to do with my husband is walking. Whether we are exploring a new neighborhood or walking out on the beach near our home in Malibu, some of my favorite moments are spent hand-in-hand, breathing in the fresh air and watching a sun set while we walk together. With every step, I feel closer to him, more free and alive, and our conversation flows freely and openly. We always finish our walks more connected, more fit, and more in love.

Of course, I also enjoy walking on my own; there's no better way to start the day than with a 15-20 minute Warrior Walk and some yoga postures to cleanse the cobwebs of sleep, oxygenate the body, recharge the energy pools, let go of the past, and start the day with a brand new, fresh start for your body, heart, mind and spirit.

When you make a commitment to do something positive for yourself, you are setting the standard for what you want in your life; this feeds over into greater success in relationships, family, career, wealth and anything you choose to create.

When you make that commitment and actually follow through with that commitment, you find a sense of strength inside you that you never knew you had. When you are faced with a challenge or obstacle, instead of triggering into the stress cycle (which drains your energy and releases the hormone cortisol, causing sugar cravings and fat storage), you find a place of calm inside of you, and you tap into that inner pool of strength available every day and every time you show up for that Warrior Walk.

You are proving to yourself, step-by-step, that you are a Warrior. "Spiritual Warrior" is a term I learned from yoga, which focuses on the concept of life not being about the battles you face on the outside, but the battles you face within: your own inner demons and the obstacles that your mind creates. It is the place inside of us all, where we overcomefear of failure or any fear of judgment from others. Nothing can stop you when you show up, take that first step and prove to yourself that you deserve it, and you can have it!

Take my hand and walk with me into a better body, a happier life, with more fun to be had every day.

> *"The journey of a thousand miles begins with a single step"*
>
> —Ancient Chinese Proverb

Keep walking!

*Andréa Albright*

Natural Weight Loss Expert
Yoga Teacher
Weight Loss Success Story (10+ years)

# Contents

| | | |
|---|---|---|
| **Introduction** | | i |
| **CHAPTER 1** | The Evolution of Walking | 1 |
| **CHAPTER 2** | The Science of Walking for Improved Health and Greater Weight Loss | 15 |
| **CHAPTER 3** | The Warrior's Walk | 30 |
| **CHAPTER 4** | Power In Your Stride | 35 |
| **CHAPTER 5** | The Warrior Walking Routines | 43 |
| **CHAPTER 6** | Conclusion | 59 |

# Introduction

The setting: New Year's Eve, 2011. Hudson Hotel Bar in Manhattan, New York City, New York.

In short, you are somewhere you really don't belong. A good friend insisted that you tag along with him and his girlfriend for New Year's Eve festivities; it was clearly more of a "sympathy" invite than anything. You had no plans and no date to speak of.

"Come on Ed, you will have a blast! The Hudson is so swank."

At this point, you will feel bad if you turn him down—he will imagine you in your grungy, ground-level apartment, sitting on your ancient olive and goldenrod plaid couch (courtesy of goodwill) in your stained, gray sweats, drinking Miller Lite and stuffing your face with piece after piece of a Supreme Tombstone pizza.

You should get out more, but, you don't belong in Manhattan on New Year's Eve. You work hard at ignoring the reservations you have about joining your friends and decide to go. You find a baggy, button-up shirt, with a scrolling cobalt pattern that will cover the top of your brown corduroy pants. Oh, the brown cords—the only pair of real pants that you can squeeze into these days, and luckily the baggy shirt will cover up the ugly way your stomach punches out of the top of the waistband.

The taxi drops you off at Columbus Circle, and you want to run away, but your friend spots you. You walk to the Hudson together, and three of you ascend the escalators to the Hudson Hotel Bar. You are engulfed in glimmering green light that sharpens the lovely features of every face in the bar, making each person look distinctive.

You are still horribly uncomfortable, and to make things worse, your friend showed up wearing a tie and dress pants. His girl is dressed to the nines and gorgeous. You are determined to make the most of this, no matter how awkward you feel—and a vodka tonic with two limes goes a long way in helping you feel mildly comfortable.

Midnight is approaching, and your friend's girl keeps making a "big to-do" about a midnight kiss. As the last minutes of 2011 evaporate into the night, you see an interesting shift in the room; the party goers have migrated slowly into precise pairs—almost as if there is a magnetic force pulling certain people together. This entire scene, these lovely parings of all shapes, sizes and colors, makes you very aware of being solo. You were already uncomfortable with the night, and while you aren't the only single body left in the room, on all sides of you couples stand close together.

You are observing all of this with a lump in your throat, and your eyes stop on an interesting girl across the room. She is dressed in an empire-waisted black dress, with wine colored tights, and chunky black ankle boots. She has horn-rimmed glasses that match her tights, and her dark brown hair is in two pig tales. She intrigues you!

The Fairy God Mother of New Year's Eve waved her wand, and all the sparkling dresses and sharp black pants swirled across the room, each linking with an enchanted partner. Yet, she forgot you, and she forgot this lovely girl, and you need the magic most of all.

Because there is no magic to be found, you will have to chuck your nervousness and just man up if you want a happy ending to your evening.

Make your way, right now, across the room to the girl with the pigtails and glasses. Only two minutes left until midnight, you need to move, but you remember again, what you are wearing and how you feel about how you look. A lead pit forms in your stomach.

You search deep within for even an ounce of confidence.

"One minute until midnight," yells a leggy blond in a silver mini-dress in the center of the room. You look harder at the pretty girl with the wine-colored glasses—you try to muster the resolve to cross the room and say hi to her; you want to kiss her, but that thought is frightening. You'll walk up, say hello, look deep into her eyes and lean in for a quick, casual kiss. You play this scene over in your head in a fast-forward mode, 15 times in a half minute.

The whole room starts counting down, "10-9." You look hard at your feet, hoping one foot will move.

"8-7-6." The girl with the glasses stands alone, playing with the striped straw in her drink.

"5-4." You notice that your knuckles have turned white from holding your drink so tight—you can't move.

"3-2." Your friend and his girl have moved in, noses touching, and you are still frozen.

"1!—Happy New Year!"

Kisses cascade around the room, followed by hollers and whoops of excitement filling the bar, the sound nearly cacophonous.

You missed it! Your moment, your opportunity, the chance to do something daring, allare gone. Your self-loathing and weak confidence have paralyzed you once again. This is not the first time, and it surely won't be the last. This moment is raw and bright red, a kick in the face. You decide, in 2012 something has to change!

No, having a girl to kiss at the stroke of midnight is not life changing, but it was a good opportunity to step outside of your dark, mopey box. You are sick and tired of standing still while your life passes you by. The way you feel about your weight and appearance have arrested your development as a human being, and more than anything, you want to look and feel healthy, with a simple confidence that equips you for getting out in the world and doing anything you desire.

The new year is the perfect time for making a commitment to change. Every January 1st, the majority of people resolve to lose weight, but resolutions are a tricky thing. The expectation attached to a resolution makes for a huge high of energy when we begin on that first day of January, but we suffer a discouraging crash when we can't keep up with the unrealistic promises we've made to ourselves.

Months after this New Year's Eve incident, you still play it over and over in your head, and it haunts you. You desperately want to change, but where do you begin? You have probably tried every weight loss gimmick imaginable—diet pills, powders, expensive weight-loss programs, and "insane" exercise routines. You have picked up this book because you are looking for a way to change your life. I am here to tell you that I can help you change your body and your health, but you must commit to altering your life (for the better) forever.

My walking workout will change your life, no matter your age, what shape you are in or how many times you have failed to lose weight.

This story reminds me of myself, when I was 62 pounds overweight and unhealthy, at the ripe old age of 30. I lacked that same confidence, because I felt awful about the way I looked. I was trapped in a vicious cycle of self-loathing, and I couldn't break free.

Whether it's ten pounds or a hundred pounds, everyone struggles to lose weight at some point. You may have started college and packed on the expected "freshman 15." For others, your metabolism caught up with you as you got older. Medications can cause weight gain. Sometimes the issue is a sedentary job or home life, or you may have no idea why you struggle with weight loss. Whatever the reason, it doesn't matter!

No matter what your reasons were for purcashing this book, my simple and straight-forward walking system is for everybody. Regardless of your current weight and shape, I can help you get lean and healthy. I guarantee that you'll see concrete results. When you get to the other side, you'll not only have the body you've always dreamed of, but the tools to maintain your body and health. How can I guarantee this? I use this same program.

Let's make it easy to tie your shoes again. Let's make it easy to get out of bed. Let's end this lifelong quest for the right exercise program, right now. You've found it. I changed from a fast food binger to a warrior using the "secret program" I outline in this book. My program is simple, you can do it at home, and you'll see results almost immediately. So join me on a journey to health; I will guide you through my program, and we will change your life forever!

# Chapter 1

## The Evolution of Walking

Imagine a bright June day in the late 90s. The sun is not quite as hot as it will be later in the summer, but it still beats down forcefully on a quaint suburban street. In the distance, you hear a lawnmower or maybe a dog barking. Children laugh at a nearby playground, enjoying those first few days of summer vacation.

On this quaint street, a man stands out in front of his house with a faint smile upon his face. It's the kind of smile that only a perfect summer day can produce. It's the kind of smile that says "At this very moment, I have not a care in the world." He stands there, hose in hand, watering the lawn in a crisp polo shirt and khaki shorts. His hair is swept back from his face with the je ne sais quoi of the well-to-do homeowner, and his freshly washed sports car gleams in the driveway.

This man is not me.

The man cocks his head to the side, listening intently. Faintly, above the noise of the lawnmower and the dog and the playing children, he hears a sound that he's never heard before: a sort of grunting, plodding sound. It's sort of a wet, rhythmic sound, *squish slosh, squish slosh*. Even worse, it's a sound that's growing more and more prominent in this quiet suburban neighborhood. Suddenly, over the gentle crest of the hill on which this picturesque home sits, a mountain of a man appears.

Drenched in sweat, the newcomer slowly heaves his bulk up the side of the hill. He wears a tank top, soaked through entirely with sweat, and gym shorts that are a size too large for him. He has to hold them up with his free hand, while the other hand holds a portable CD player. His shoes are the source of the rhythmic sound, and they look similarly soaked through with sweat. They also look like they're about to burst open with all the strain this man has put on them today. Breathing heavily, this new apparition reaches the top of the hill, comes to a stop in the middle of the road, and rests his hands on his knees.

This sweating mass of man, this behemoth of blubber--this is me fifteen years ago, shortly after I began walking for my health.

I straighten up, ready to continue on my way. Out of the corner of my eye, I notice the man watering his lawn and staring at me, not unkindly. In fact, he seems almost sympathetic, watching me surmount this latest obstacle in my walk that day. Proudly, with the self-assurance of a man working hard to better himself, I raise my hand to wave at him. He nods and waves back at me. "Hot day out, eh?" he asks me, smiling with encouragement.

"You have no idea," I respond. He laughs and gives me a quick salute, and down the hill I go.

• • •

Fifteen years ago, I began walking to improve my fitness. I was obese and finally fed up with it. I was carrying around an additional 62 pounds of blubber that my body simply could not handle. *62 pounds*. The idea is almost inconceivable to me now. I don't even really know how it got that bad to begin with.

If you've never been that overweight, you can't begin to understand the toll that everyday activity takes on your body. Imagine just walking around, doing your daily errands or going to work, except that somebody strapped a small child or a large dog to your back, and you can't get rid of it. You aren't very good at getting out of bed, and walking down stairs is a craps shoot, because you can't see your feet. At all.

Of course, if you have been or currently are overweight, you understand all too well what I'm talking about. I was disease-ridden and frail, unable to enjoy my life or hobbies, all this at the ripe old age of thirty-one. I decided that I needed to make a change. The prospect of another year trapped in that decrepit body shook me to my core. The time to reinvent my life was now. I talked to my doctor, who hemmed and hawed a lot about my weight in general. He was overly enthusiastic when I told him I was considering exercise. That afternoon I went home, grabbed some comfortable shoes, and started walking for my health.

Walking, at the time, was not my exercise of choice—it was literally the only exercise I was capable of doing. Believe me, I could hear the world groan with protest after every step I took. Even so, walking was an ordeal. Just traipsing around my suburban neighborhood left me gasping for air, as if I had scaled Everest. My feet ached from carrying so much extra weight, and I had never sweat so much in my life. I had no idea, however, that the trail I was blazing was one that would change, not just my level of fitness, but also the way I viewed health and vitality forever. Nowadays, thanks to walking and the increased shape it's put me in, I feel even younger than I did back then.

Walking. Chances are, you do it every day without even thinking twice about it. It's one of the first things you learn as a child, and it's one of the abilities that humans are most loathe to relinquish. What's more, walking is a powerful tool for weight loss, when used correctly. Whether you're just going from the parking lot into your office building or taking a leisurely stroll after a long day, you're utilizing one of the best methods your body has for exercise, without even realizing it.

The most common question I get when it comes to the cardio portion of my training is, "How often do you run?" (Feel free to substitute run for any other high-intensity, high-impact exercise). My response is always, of course, "I never run. I walk. Period."

My answer should be recorded to save my breath.

I know, I know. I'm sure you've heard people scoff at walking for exercise. Maybe you've even done it yourself. Walking? Well that's a waste of momentum at best, and an old man's hobby at worst.

Walking is what golfers do between holes, and there's certainly no shortage of fat golfers out there. "Real men" (and women!) engage in "real exercise": running, cycling, mountain biking, swimming, football, rugby, full-contact kickboxing, these are the activities you've always envisioned for yourself, but never have actually done.

What most people don't understand is that you don't even have to do *any* of these more "productive" exercises in order to get in shape. I once had the same mistaken notions, before walking for health reasons completely changed my level of physique. Today, in spite of my single-digit body fat levels and competition bodybuilder physique, I still nearly exclusively walk for cardio and weight management.

People always look shocked and are full of disbelief when I tell them about walking. Our culture has become so ingrained with the idea that high-intensity exercise and being in shape are synonymous; because of this, people assume that I also must have attained my body inthrough some intense workout plan. They picture me spending all my time in the gym, running for hours at a time, only stopping to jump rope or do some crunches. After all, that's how all men get in shape, right?

Running to get in shape is such a foreign idea to me. Think of all the damage that you're doing to your joints in the long run. Sure, you might be in shape for a couple of years (or even longer, if you're dedicated to it). However, you're going to be in for a whole host of side effects ten or twenty years down the road. Getting into shape so that you can live longer is useless if you then have to spend all of those years with pain in your knees and hips, especially if you could get the same workout through a much less damaging exercise. In fact, most high-intensity exercise follows that pattern. You're getting results slightly faster, maybe (some studies even dispute that), but at what cost?

I'm not going to lie to you. I'm not going to tell you that this is going to be easy. It's not even going to be "sort of easy." If you walk down this road with me, you're going to work hard. You're going to push yourself harder than you've probably ever pushed yourself before. Do you know that reserve of energy deep in your gut that lets you push your body for one or two seconds longer than it thinks it can go? You are going to access that reserve every single day. If you're willing to listen, I'm going to teach you the basics of how to live a healthy and fulfilling life.

I know you have doubts, but don't worry. I know that it sounds too good to be true. Walking? Well, what's offensive about that? Exercise means suffering. Exercise means pain. All those high-intensity workouts I listed above, that's exercise. You have to beat your body into submission to do those, right? Believe me, I've been in your position before, and I know how this sounds.

This is no ordinary walking, however. As I'll show you later in this book, you will be working hard. The two S's of your everyday workout—sweating and soreness—will definitely come into play here. I know you don't believe me yet, but this program is going to wear you out even after you've reached your peak levels of fitness.

What's more, I love walking. I love its simplicity; I love the sense of peace and well being it gives me to take a long walk, whether I'm out in the sun or indoors. I love the convenience, in spite of doing most of my walking these days in the gym on a treadmill. I love its effectiveness, without the drain on my workout recovery or strain on my joints. I love coming home after a good walk and feeling that dull burn in my muscles that lets me know I had a good workout.

I preach a simple gospel: do what you love to do, and you will keep on doing it. It's an easy gospel to remember, but surprisingly few people put it into practice. Instead, they choose their weight loss plans based on what others choose. You know these people; they're the ones who bounce between diets like they're playing pinball, or run for a few weeks every year before giving up again. They don't like what they're doing, and that's their first hurdle when it comes to losing the weight.

Don't follow their example. You need to pick something and stick to it, or else you will never get anywhere at all. The person who stretches themselves in a thousand directions follows through on none of them. Choose something you already enjoy, even if it's just moderate enjoyment, so that you won't want to give up later when it gets hard (and it's going to get hard). I love walking; therefore, I never have to worry about falling off the "bandwagon."

What could be more natural than walking? As I said, you already do it every day. All that this book teaches you is how to walk for your health instead of simply walking for transportation. It's like learning to drive a finely-tuned race car instead of commuting through traffic every day. What's the point of owning a nice car if you don't keep it in peak condition? Adding intensity and regularity to your walking routine will quickly transform you into a fat-burning machine. It's low-intensity, high-efficiency exercise for the masses.

Better yet, there aren't any catches, no "gotcha" moment at the end, no life-impacting injuries or high-priced exercise equipment. You can work at it wherever you are and whatever your financial situation. I'm not trying to sell you any expensive equipment; I just want to help you, because I've seen what a huge difference this program can make. Keep walking, and all you're going to receive are some worn out shoes, admiring glances and a toned body.

I've heard people say that they're afraid walking will take too long in producing visible results. You want results, and you want them now! How will you notice any reasonable progress if walking is such a low-intensity workout?

I'm telling you, it will be impossible for you to not notice the results, even after a relatively short period of time. Walking burns more fat *exclusively* than any other single activity. Sure, that is a loaded statement. Obviously, a competitive triathlete would disagree with it, making a case for hours of cycling, swimming, running, and occasional trips to the emergency room.

Yet, it's an argument they rarely win. Walking, when done as instructed in this book, will keep you under what's known as the *lactate threshold*. This is the point at which your body switches from burning primarily fatty acids for fuel to burning sugar for fuel.

Correct me if I'm wrong, but you probably don't care about burning *sugar*. Sugar is a great fuel source for the body during times of exertion. In fact, that's why the body switches over to burning it so eagerly. Sugar has high energy content, and is pretty easy for the body to access. Even in the best of us, however, it's in short supply—about 800 grams worth in a 300-pound bodybuilder, to give you an idea. The rest of us store 200-400 grams of sugar in the muscles, and perhaps 100 grams in the liver.

Fat, on the other hand, is ample. Overstocked, marked down, and primed to move. You couldn't pay people enough to take this stuff off your hands. You have pounds and pounds of fat on your body, versus "grams" of sugar (stored as glycogen in your liver and muscles, along with blood sugar). There's no bag marked "sugar" just hanging around in that flab around your waist, waiting to be burned. No, all of that is fat, through and through.

Sugar is easy to burn. All you need is to get your heart rate up enough to where your breathing becomes labored, and presto: you're burning a boatload of sugar. Then your body doesn't switch back to burning fat again until it's burned through all the sugar it can find. That process can take quite a while. Fat is not so easy to burn, now is it?

Doesn't it make more sense to concentrate on an activity that, as exercise goes, is virtually a pure fat-burner? I certainly think so. After all, it's not the sugar in your body that's making you feel self-conscious.

That's not to say this book is a license to eat sugars. The body's energy processes are a bit more complicated than that. All that sugar you eat actually does get broken down and turned into fat eventually, which is just as bad. While we may not store much sugar in our body as sugar, we certainly put the pounds on by eating it. Don't go eating that entire chocolate cake just because Jon Benson (that's me) told you that your body doesn't store sugar. You are what you eat, and in this case, eating a plateful of sugary concoctions means you are going to put on the pounds.

My point is that we should burn the fat you already have instead of getting rid of sugar that your body is going to use up anyway. Your body is going to burn off that sugar eventually whether you do high-intensity exercise or not. However, it takes a lot more work to burn off those fat reserves. What I'm proposing is that we do low-intensity exercise, exclusively focusing on getting rid of those pesky fat reserves that have us wearing our shirts at the beach. The sugars will sort themselves out.

Walking is one of the most pure, unadulterated fat-burning exercises you can do. Even moderate-paced walking burns fat, nearly exclusively. However, we want to get results that you can notice, and moderate-paced walking just isn't going to do it. We want to speed things up a bit, so the walking routines covered in this book will look to do just that. Just make sure that in the process you don't end up running instead of walking quickly.

The reason, again, is the lactate threshold. Once your body perceives strenuous exertion, it shifts to burning sugar. There are quite a few theories behind why this simple process occurs, but the one I favor is evolutionary in origin.

Have you ever considered why you store fat? Chances are, you've never even thought about it before. It's just one of those things that seem beyond questions, like July 4th and grandma's apple pie, or black shoes and brown socks. If I asked you right now why you store fat, you may be tempted to answer, "Because God hates me," or "Because I eat pizza at midnight," or "Because someone has a voodoo doll with my likeness, and they're having a really good laugh right about now." While all of those things may be correct in some part, there is a more basic reason for why humans store fat—and a very good reason at that.

Without the ability to store fat, you would not be reading this book, nor would I be around to write it. Storing fat was crucial for our cave-dwelling ancestors' survival.[i] Food was a bit more difficult to come by in those days and had to be hunted or scavenged, instead of cultivated. There was no steady supply. If you finally managed to take down a wooly mammoth, well, eating the entire beast as soon as possible probably seemed like a very good idea back then (the equivalent is done today at your neighborhood fast food joint, and it's never a good idea). After all, you didn't want other predators to steal the precious meat from you, and you never knew when that next wooly would make an appearance (or how accurate your aim would be if and when he did).

Come wintertime, any plant-based foods (fruits, vegetables, and primitive grains) were almost impossible to find in the frozen tundra of the savannah. The bodies of our ancestors, at least those who survived, were often ravaged. Survival in this frozen wasteland would have been absolutely impossible for all but a select few, had it not been for one brilliant design.

*Love Handles.* Saddlebags. Basketball Bellies. Wave-Twice Triceps. Cottage Cheese Thighs. More Cushion For The Pushin'.

All of these things that we love to hate, these scourges of modern humankind, were the product of nature creating a knapsack of energy reserves to keep us functioning efficiently. Without it, we would have gone the way of the dodo bird during the harsh winters, too hungry and malnourished to do anything but wile away the days until extinction. With it, we had the fuel needed to chase down that wooly mammoth, stray rabbit or that pesky Bambi critter (Note: I'm being facetious, just in case there are any paleontologists interested in walking). The point is, fat storage gave humanity had a chance to survive.

Fat was used during long walks to hunt or forage, as well as for spurts of intense 'exercise', such as getting your butt out of the way of any fastapproaching tiger. Fat was used in the place of carbohydrates, because, big surprise, there were very little carbohydrates, at least not enough for your body to burn reliably all day long. Sugar became our body's luxury energy source, used for strenuous exercise until it was gone, after which the body switched back to burning fat.

Fat was, and still is, a very dense, very powerful fuel source. Thanks to this evolutionary pattern of development, your heart runs almost exclusively on fat. Your brain is primarily composed out of the same 3-letter swear word. Without fat, the part of your brain that decodes these little squiggles into actual letters, and then words, would not function. Cholesterol, vilified in the media, is actually a mother hormone, responsible for the creation of little baby hormones with not-so-cute little names (testosterone, androstendione, and other European-sounding monikers). Fat, whether ingested from animals or stored and ready-to-use, allowed us to live to eat another day.

That other day has arrived, and we no longer need this lifesaver hanging around our waistline like a rubbery, ugly, and detestable life preserver. Food is available in the masses, advertised on TV, on the bus, on billboards, on the radio. Gigantic supermarkets filled with row upon row of cream-filled cookies, pasta, energy drinks, frozen burritos, and (if you live in certain states) alcoholic beverages. It's enough to intimidate a person into submission and induce a life of overeating, followed by stressful weight-loss diets. It's enough to cause normal men and women to enter into a hateful relationship with that dirty ol' rascal, fat.

We've evolved. Our food sources have evolved. Our fat stores have not. They're the same machines that have been chugging along for thousands of years now. While evolution can be a great tool, and it definitely saved our skins back when humanity could have died out, it's also a slow process. We've yet to adapt to the idea of having too much food.

Therefore, we have to work hard at burning fat. That requires three specific things: walking (with planned "spurts" of running from tigers), a diet lower in carbohydrates and resistance-bearing exercise. Remember, they carried their wooly mammoths back to the cave. That required muscle, and so do you.

Walking (or, more specifically, "interval walking") replicates the motion of our ancestors. They were not long-distance runners; despite the respect given to marathon runners, both historically and in the modern day, this type of exercise is hardly standard to humankind's development. Ancestral humans walked long distances at a brisk pace, occasionally interrupted by flashes of sheer terror when sprinting was required. When that tiger came around, it was either run or be eaten.

This blend of long, brisk walks and short bursts of higher blood-volume exercise, steadily utilized the fat stores in ancestral humans. It preserved the very limited supply of glycogen and kept their calorie-burning muscle mass intact. It made them lean—not skinny, but toned. Yes, toned. The same body-type that you've been pursuing for years now came naturally to your ancestors, simply due to their lifestyles. There's no reason that you can't have the same body. All you have to do is embrace what your body evolved to do years ago, instead of trying to force it into shape.

Unfortunately, this book doesn't come with any tigers. Of course, there's no way to *really* recreate the environment of our ancestors, and I also know that sprinting comes with almost as many stigmas as walking does—long hot days spent out on the track for gym class in those silly shorts, or (gulp) running suicides on that squeaky basketball court.

Fortunately for your once-wounded pride, sprinting in the truest sense of the term is not required in this program. Remember, I started exercising when I was so overweight that I could only handle walking.

I take pride in the fact that this program being so forgiving to newcomers, and I understand that sprinting automatically scares people off. However, sprinting would defeat our goal of weight-loss through low-intensity, high-efficiency exercises. While it may be efficient and mimic what our ancestors did, it can also cause problems with your joints if performed incorrectly. Instead, I've opted to preserve your body (and sanity) by merely asking for one to two-minute intervals of "walking climbs." Don't worry if you don't know what that means. All will be explained in the coming chapters.

I understand if you still have some concerns. You mayy feel that walking is not as easy to tell your friends about as some other exercises. It's easy to say that you dropped two pants sizes by running or by fighting off bears, but walking? Well, maybe your friends are going to look at you a bit weird if you say that.

Personally, I think that worry is all in your head. First of all, finishing this book will provide you with all the science behind walking for your health, helping you to explain the program to skeptics. I'm not just explaining to you how to walk for your health, I'm explaining *why* you should walk for your health. Both of those aspects are important when it comes to weight loss. You'll be thankful for the extra motivation later on, when the going gets tough.

On top of all that, your results will soon speak for themselves. You'll be looking and feeling so good that you won't care anymore what people think of your walking regimen. Even your most skeptical friends will have to admit they were wrong when they see the kind of results you're getting. Within no time, they'll be coming to you, begging for the secret workout ingredient that led to such a toned body. Of course, you're free to tell them, or not tell them, about my program as you wish.

It's an even easier sell when I tell you that, with the right equipment (meaning just a treadmill), you can do all of this at home if you choose to do so. It requires no expensive gym membership, no hot sun, no curious glances from the neighbors, no time spent commuting to and from where you want to work out. No, all of this furious fat-burning can be done in the quiet, air-conditioned (or heated) comfort of your own home. Flip the TV on while you work out, or maybe some of your favorite tunes. Then, when you're done, just pop into the shower and come out feeling refreshed again. Except for the soreness (and it's a good soreness, believe me), it's like you didn't even work out! For my money, working out at home is one of the best experiences you can have.

On the other hand, don't be afraid to get out in the sun and strut on those streets. There's something to be said about walking around the neighborhood, quietly taking in the sights after a hard day at work, or early in the morning before everyone's awake. An outdoor walk can be inspiring and peaceful, if you choose the right spot. Try finding a nice hiking trail, or something with a lot of vertical climbs. That will be the best spot to emulate what I would have you do on a treadmill.

Whatever the method you choose, I'm already proud of you. As they always say, the first step is admitting that there is a problem. You can't take action until you know that there's an action to be taken. Maybe you're a seasoned veteran of various workout and diet programs, or maybe you've only recently decided that it's time to lose weight. Maybe this is a result of your latest New Year's Resolution, or concern about your latest doctor visit. Maybe you feel like you're being out-paced, whether by your grandkids or the world in general. Maybe you just want to go to the beach without feeling awkward.

Regardless, you've already made it farther in your quest than a lot of people ever do, by looking for a reliable, real-world method for losing weight. I know that people come to their weight loss realization through a number of different avenues, but at the end of the day we're all in this together. You're going to hear me say this a lot in this book, but I just want to say it now, up front, and before we've really gotten into the meat of the issue: I believe that you can do this. I believe that you can lose this weight.

I know what you're thinking. "But Jon, you've never met me. How could you know?"

I know because everyone has the power to do this. Everyone has the power to make a positive change in their lifestyle. My program is very technical and will test your willpower. I have made it as easy as possible for anyone with a little self-determination to make it through. I know that you can lose this weight, because you are where I was fifteen years ago.

I've already seen the benefits of this program. Now I'm going to try and prove those same benefits to you. It's sort of a "pay-it-forward" type of program. I was lucky enough to stumble upon this routine all those years ago when I needed help, and now I want you to have the same help. You deserve a weight loss program that works, because nobody should have to be overweight if they are willing to put in the effort. You deserve to have that body you've always dreamed of, and as long as you keep reading this book and take the steps I prescribe, that dream body is within your grasp.

What about the other two parts of the picture, you ask? If you want to put all three pieces of the puzzle together, you will need to pick up two other books. The first is, *The Every Other Day Diet*, a fun, lifestyle-friendly diet plan. Think about the principles we've talked about so far in terms of exercising: our bodies evolved a certain way. The closer we can come to emulating those ancestral patterns of behavior in the modern world, the healthier we're going to feel. *The Every Other Day Diet* follows the same tactic, integrating aspects of our caveman lineage into an exciting, easy-to-follow formula. Even better, this diet plan makes use of frequent "Feed Meals," allowing you to eat your favorite foods throughout the week.

Also pick up *7 Minute Muscle*. While *Walk Your Way Thin* is a great exercise regimen to get you started on the path to fitness, it's only the first step. You will be toned and in better shape after just a short time using this program. However, *7 Minute Muscle* is another set of my personal short-but-intense workouts designed to shape muscle faster and more efficiently than ever. Walking will help you lose the weight and slim down, but resistance training will help you bulk back up (this time, with muscle) and give you the strength you've always wanted.

With all three books in hand, you will quickly be in the best shape of your life. "Eat right and exercise," is age-old advice, but my books will break it all down into manageable, decisive steps and keep you on the right path. If I can lose 62 pounds of fat with this program, anything is possible.

i    Barrett, Deirdre. *Waistland: The (R)evolutionary Science behind Our Weight and Fitness Crisis.* New York: W.W. Norton & Co., 2007.

# Chapter 2

# The Science of Walking for Improved Health and Greater Weight Loss

The doctor's office is shiny and bright, perfectly ordered and obviously cared for. I sit in one of a dozen identical chairs, absentmindedly flipping through the latest version of Life or Us Weekly or one of the other stereotypical doctor's office magazines. Some celebrity graces the cover, looking toned and thin. I think she was in a movie recently, and I try to figure out which one. Something about a sinking ship, maybe…I stare through the pages of the magazine, eyes unfocused and barely open. In my head, a song by the latest boy band plays on repeat.

The doctor comes out, wiping his hands on his spotless white jacket. "Come on back, Mr. Benson," he says with a smile and a handshake. I notice there actually is a small spot on his lapel, maybe of ketchup or hot sauce. He leads me down a labyrinth of featureless corridors. Just a few months ago, this walk would have left me gasping for air. Now? Well, I'm not exactly sprinting down the hall, but my heart also doesn't feel like it's going to burst out of my chest like a creature in some science fiction film.

In fact, I feel pretty incredible. I've been dieting and exercising for nearly half a year, and my whole body can feel the difference. Miles and miles of walking have left me in better shape than I've been in for years. First, I had to go out and buy a new belt to keep my pants up, and then I recently had to go and buy new pants entirely. My shirts are like an ocean of cotton at this point; soon I'll need to replace all of those, too. When I'm out on the town, my feet no longer hurt (or at least not as much as they used to), and I can walk both further and faster than I ever could have dreamed when I started my routine. My confidence has skyrocketed. Not only is the exercise releasing a semi-constant stream of endorphins into my blood, but I look and feel better than ever before. I feel like a new man.

"Up on the scale," the doctor says. I glare at the scale, my long-hated enemy. For years I have done battle with this fearsome foe, always coming out on the losing end. I watched over time as my weight went continued on an upward trend, feeling helpless and beaten down. This time, though, things are different.

I hop on the scale and stare down over the ever-shrinking remnant of my gut. The needle swings back and forth for a second before coming slowly to rest.

"Much better," the doctor murmurs. "Much, much better."

• • •

It's not just the weight loss that my doctor is excited about. While weight loss in and of itself is a great goal for your physical comfort and mental well-being, it also is important for your long-term health. Let's take a look at what our friend science has to say about walking. Can it really be that helpful to our bodies? I know that despite all my talk of ancestral humanity and natural evolution in the last chapter, you're still probably skeptical. Fortunately for me (and you!), scientists worldwide have demonstrated quite a few correlations between moderate walking and improved health.

Sure, many of you just want to walk your way thin. Perhaps you just want to figure out a way to lose that last pesky ten pounds, or maybe you're like I once was and need to lose a ton of weight. Either way, you might be interested to know that walking does much more than shed excess body fat. In the studies cited in the coming chapters, you will learn how walking may reduce the risk factors for numerous chronic diseases, including heart disease, diabetes, stroke, cancer and even the common cold. It's been linked to improved mood, overall mental health, and reduced risk of cognitive impairment. For many, it is a welcome stress-relief, and some even find spiritual wellness though regular walking. All it requires is a little effort, literally.

In this chapter, I've collected a number of scientific papers that prove how good walking is, not just for weight loss, but for preventing diseases and reshaping your entire lifestyle. That way, you don't just have to take my word for it.

As you read along, do note that many clinical studies are gender-specific for the purpose of statistical analysis. This does not mean that the clinical results discussed indicate the benefits of regular walking are gender-specific. Look at it this way: unless you do not have a body part specifically indicated in the experiment (heart, lungs, legs, etc.), it is likely you could benefit just as well as the gender studied.

## Lung Health

Many people are familiar with the correlation between aerobic activity and lung health. That seems self-explanatory, right? Well you may be surprised to know that you don't have to run marathons, or run at all, for that matter, to improve your lung health. In Barcelona, Spain, The Municipal Unit of Medical Investigation studied the effects of walking on patients with Chronic Obstructive Pulmonary Disease (COPD).[ii] This disease is an unfortunate combination of emphysema and chronic bronchitis, which obstructs airflow and requires frequent hospitalization. Common wisdom often dictated that patients with COPD avoid strenuous exercise so as to not trigger an attack. What did the team of researchers find?

They actually discovered that the exact opposite was true. Common wisdom, in this case, was entirely mistaken. As the study said, "to our knowledge, this is the first study to show that patients with COPD who perform a relatively high level of physical activity in their daily life have a substantially reduced risk of readmission due to exacerbation." What was this relatively high level of physical activity? The study required that the patients walk for about an hour a day. This reduced their chance of hospitalization by 50% over patients who were not active.

One hour of walking per day, not even at a strenuous pace. Just that moderate amount of time spent walking provides a measurable increase in lung health. With *Walk Your Way Thin*, where we'll be combining a brisker walk with periods of more strenuous activity, your lung health should improve quickly and noticeably.

## Diabetes

Two-thirds of Americans are overweight or obese. Americans are more likely than ever to develop Type 2 Diabetes, and this has caused some medical professionals to hypothesize that the current generation of American children could actually have shorter life expectancies than their parents.[iii] If so, this would be the first decline in life expectancy that America has experienced in decades.

Diabetes is hard enough on its own, but mismanagement of a diabetic condition can be even worse. We're looking at a future with high rates of amputations, impotence, kidney failure and blindness if we can't beat this spate of Type 2 Diabetes. That's a mighty bleak future ahead of us, if trends continue on their projected path. So, how can walking help battle this emerging epidemic?

The Graduate School of Public Health at the University of Pittsburgh found that walking **for just 30 minutes a day** reduced the risk of developing diabetes for both men and women who were overweight and even slightly helped those who were not overweight. Physical activity not only reduces an individual's risk for diabetes through weight loss, but through exercise itself.

As the study points out, "Beyond the effect of activity on body mass and composition, physical activity may reduce the risk for Type 2 diabetes directly through improvements in insulin sensitivity. However, a large portion of the effect of physical activity in decreasing insulin resistance is short lived and may last only a few days."[iv] Thus, a consistent and planned exercise routine can help lower the risk of diabetes in an individual even if they aren't losing any weight and their body mass index (BMI) stays the same. Since you will be sloughing off weight during this program, this may not be as applicable to you. However, you should know that walking will help you prevent Type 2 Diabetes, no matter what form that prevention takes.

The Diabetes Prevention Program, a large-scale and government-funded research study, produced similar results.[v] Overweight participants with high blood sugar who made even moderate changes in eating habits and walked an average of 30 minutes a day over the course of a year cut their risk of developing diabetes by half. The authors of the study went on to claim that "it should also be possible to delay or prevent the development of complications, substantially reducing the individual and public health burden of diabetes."

Think about that for a second. Changing your lifestyle even in this small way could have a significant impact on whether you succumb to this growing epidemic or not. Personally, I'd bet that Type 2 Diabetes is something you'd like to avoid. Well, science says that you can, and I'm here to help you do it.

The onset of gestational diabetes in pregnancy is also becoming commonplace in America. Once again, regular walking can provide quantifiable benefits. The results of a collaborative study were published in the American Journal of Epidemiology, Volume 159. The study "assessed risk of gestational diabetes mellitus in relation to weekly energy expenditure on recreational physical activity, which integrates intensity and the amount of time spent exercising during pregnancy and during the year before pregnancy."[vi] In other words, it looked at how much exercise expectant mothers did prior to their child's birth, and then saw if that had any effect on gestational diabetes. The results showed that expecting mothers who participated in 4.2 or more hours of recreational activity a week reduced their gestational diabetes mellitus risk *by 76%.*

That's an incredible statistic, and really shows the effect that walking can have on your life whether you're an expectant mother or not. Obviously, we are meant for physical activity. The effects of even moderate exercise are significant and measurable, and the benefits don't stop there.

## Bone Health

One of the longest on-going clinical studies in women's health, The Nurses' Health Study, has followed over 120,000 nurses since 1976. With that many scrubs in active participation, I'm sure you're not surprised to find this is one of the largest-scale studies on women's health to-date. The series of studies investigate risk factors for major chronic diseases such as breast cancer, colon cancer and cardiovascular disease. The studies have also closely monitored risk of hip fracture, and loss of cognitive functioning.

In terms of bone health, The Nurses' Health Study answers succinctly and definitively: "More physical activity, including walking, reduces risk of hip fracture."[vii] I couldn't ask for a better endorsement for walking if I tried.

## Cancer

According to this same study, "Physical activity (more than 3 hours per week) reduces risk" for developing breast cancer and colon cancer also. The research from the Nurses' Health Study provided proof that walking reduces the risk of breast cancer, colon cancer, coronary heart disease, stroke, hip fracture, and loss of cognitive functioning.

Additionally, The MacMillan Cancer Support Organization analyzed and complied data from numerous clinical studies, medical journals and experts in their recent 2011 evidence review. The in-depth summary indicated "that physical activity is associated with reduced risk of developing breast cancer." Women who exercised regularly showed decreased amounts of estrogen, high levels of which are associated with breast cancer. Finally, breast cancer patients who walked the equivalent of 150 minutes a week had a 40% lower chance of dying from their breast cancer or failed remission than the comparison group of women who lived mostly sedentary lifestyles and were typically active for less than an hour a week.

Don't worry, males, walking reduces your risk of cancer, as well. As the MacMillan study says regarding cancer prevention through exercise, "There is evidence of a dose-response (i.e. the more physical activity, the greater any benefits). Even a modest amount of exercise is beneficial, and will see gains versus doing nothing at all."

If, heaven forbid, you are diagnosed with cancer, walking can even help your recovery. A 2010 study of cancer survivors showed that physical activity during recovery can increase energy and lessen fatigue related to treatment. The study claims that, "a small to moderate positive effect of physical activity during treatment was seen for physical activity level, aerobic fitness, muscular strength, functional quality of life, anxiety and self-esteem."[viii]

## Stroke and Heart Health

Men, while less at risk of developing breast cancer, often develop coronary issues later on in life. Walking can help with that too! The Harvard Alumni Health Study followed male graduates for 13 years, concluding that those who walked 20 kilometers (roughly 12.5 miles) or more a week significantly reduced their risk of stroke.[ix] At the rate I eventually want to get you walking (a mile every fifteen minutes) that's even *less* than half an hour of walking per day.

The Honolulu Heart Program monitored 8,000 Hawaiian men aged 45-68 for the development of cardiovascular problems and other causes of death.[x] Follow-up additions to the study monitored the walking habits of men over a 12-year period. The follow-up study found that men who participated in one hour of moderate activity a day (walking) had more than a 50% reduction in mortality rate than the men who led less active lifestyles. Researchers also found that the men who walked less than one mile a day were 2.5 times more likely to die from cancer than the men who walked two or more miles a day. Data trends also pointed to correlations between increased walking and reduced risk of cardiovascular disease and diabetes.

Again, we see that even a moderate amount of walking can improve your health in a myriad of ways, not just in terms of weight loss. If you are at all concerned with diseases, adding some physical activity to your daily routine will greatly improve your chances of preventing or surviving all kinds of problems. Even if you're not interested in diabetes or pulmonary health, I'd bet that you are definitely interested in...

## Sex

A Boston University School of Medicine Study followed the urological health of 600 men over a period of nine years.[xi] Here it is, ladies and gentlemen: walking can improve your sex life. That's right, it's a miracle. Let's break it down into layman's terms, for all you skeptics: walking improves blood flow, and increased blood flow prevents impotence, just as it prevents heart attacks. Both men and women can appreciate this added benefit.

Of course, it might also improve your sex life in ways that are less associated with blood flow. Losing all of this weight and finally getting into shape will boost not only your physical attractiveness, but also your self-confidence. You'll be feeling and looking better than ever before, allowing you to take more chances when it comes to the opposite sex. I'm not going to outright claim that walking is the best thing that could ever happen to your sex life, but it very well might be.

Maybe *that's* all the motivation you need to get out there and start walking.

## The Common Cold

A 2006 study conducted at the Fred Hutchinson Cancer Research Center investigated the link between moderate exercise and the risk of catching a cold.[xii] The data recorded included 115 inactive, overweight, postmenopausal women who began exercising an average of 30 minutes a day for one year. Conclusions drawn from the study indicated women who walked 30 minutes or more a day reduced the risk of catching a cold by 50%. How far would you go to get rid of those dreaded winter sniffles? Would you start walking for just 30 minutes a day? That seems like a small price to pay for a winter without crumpled tissues and sore throats.

## Brain Health

The brain is one of the most important parts of the body, and also one of the saddest to see decline. Aging in and of itself takes a toll on the brain over time, which is why you might not feel as sharp as you did twenty years ago. Maybe those math problems take longer than they used to, or maybe you can't finish the Sunday crossword anymore. Every doctor seems to have a method to help stave off this curse, whether it's taking up knitting or trying Sudoku. Would you believe that exercise also helps?

A 2010 collaborative study published in Frontiers in Aging Neuroscience found that walking about 40 minutes, 3 times a week, could greatly improve brain connectivity between crucial circuits that erode with age.[xiii] Fight off dementia and keep your body active! The conclusions also underline the idea that lifestyle overhauls are not necessary to see positive health changes; rather, moderate aerobic activity on a consistent basis will improve brain function.

The Radiological Society of North America conducted a study that found walking might slow down the cognitive diminution in patients with Alzheimer's disease, and even moderate cognitive impairment in pre-Alzheimer healthy adults.[xiv] Patients who walked about five miles a week maintained cognitive function at much greater rate than those who were inactive, and healthy adults needed to walk about six miles a week to maintain current cognitive function. So, if you can't remember to walk, you may be able to walk to remember.

## Depression

Walking can even make you feel better emotionally. A study conducted in 2005 by researchers at the University of Texas concluded that a single 30-minute bout of moderately-paced walking had a positive effect on the mood and well being of participants diagnosed with Major Depressive Disorder.[xv] In terms of mood boosters, walking is near instant gratification. When in self-doubt, hit the track and get back in your groove. A treadmill or urban route will do, but if possible, consider a green, outdoor option like a park or walking trail.

There must be substance behind the old cliché "step out for some fresh air." Mind, a British mental health organization sourced data from two studies conducted by the University of Essex.[xvi] They found that following an outdoor walk, 90% of the clinically depressed participants felt positive changes in self-esteem and 71% felt a decrease in both depression symptoms and tension. That's an astounding statistic for such a small lifestyle change.

## Weight Loss

We've touched on many of the astounding health benefits achievable though the act of routine walking. There's not a catch. Walking, when done consistently, will greatly improve your quality of life, both now and far down the line. By walking, you're taking control of your own health.

On the other hand, many people get into exercise for one reason and one reason only. Sure, they love the added benefits to their health, and they'll appreciate all those aspects in good time. However, most people embark on this journey to lose weight, and those are all the results they need. That mythical six-pack, washboard abdominal section is the goal here, and if the heart or brain happens to benefit in the meantime, the more the merrier.

What does science have to say? Well, it's quite obvious, really. There's no trick when it comes to walking for weight loss. In simple terms, losing weight occurs and increases as walking pace, duration, and frequency increase. But hey, you probably already knew that.

The Mayo Foundation for Medical Education and Research published "Walking for Fitness, A Step in the Right Direction," detailing how the average person burns about 400 calories in a one-hour brisk walk.[xvii] Of course, that's purely an average and may or may not apply to your current situation. Depending on your current weight and level of fitness, you could be burning more or less calories within the same amount of time as that "average." I know you're thinking. "But, Jon, 400 calories isn't that much! 400 calories barely even covers the burger I ate for lunch!" It's true, 400 calories might not sound like a lot of energy burned.

Think of it this way, though. That's 400 calories your body now doesn't store as fat. It's 400 calories that your body used to rely on during the day that are now gone. Now, to make up that 400 calories, your body has to remove it from the weight you've already put on. It needs to dip into its reserves, so to speak, in order to keep your body running throughout the day.

Our bodies were designed to move, and walking is one of the best ways to satisfy the fundamental need for physical activity. The reason we eat is to fuel that need to keep on moving. Then, we keep on moving so that, eventually, our body needs to eat again. It's a cycle, and one that needs to be put back into balance in order for us to meet our weight loss goals.

The other really interesting point from the same Mayo Foundation study is that you burn roughly 400 calories in an *intense* 20-30 minute bout of cardio. However, most of these calories are pulled from your glycogen stores, while walking draws mostly from your fat stores. Like I discussed in the introduction, we don't want to burn *sugar*. We want that pesky fat to hit the road. You should save your labor-intensive exercise time for *resistance training*, which is a far more effective long-term fat burner.

You probably noticed that all the studies I discussed in this chapter prescribed slightly different calculations concerning the recommended walking duration and frequency, depending on the resulting health benefit that was studied. It can all be confusing. "Should I walk three times a week or four? What if I want the health benefits described for two different parts of my body? What if I only want to lose weight? After all, I want to avoid that whole 'overtraining' thing that we discussed earlier!"

Don't worry. I'm here to guide you through all of that later. I've read even more studies than I've listed in this book, and taken all of that knowledge into account when I devised my three-part plan. Regardless of what your goal is, I'm going to help you reach it. I only wanted you to read the clinical information just as it was reported.

Before we continue on, however, let's look at one more study that specifically addresses the *time duration* factor. I want to show you just how small a commitment you're going to need to make every week in order to lose the weight. It's still a commitment, and it's still going to be hard, but this study goes to show you that provable and notable weight loss is attainable no matter what your situation.

A recent study conducted by the University of Miami, "Dose-Response Effect of Walking Exercise on Weight Loss. How Much is Enough?" examined the effects that two different walking durations (in combination with a diet program) had on weight loss.[xviii] Participants in the 12-week weight loss intervention study were ethnically diverse, overweight, premenopausal women who strictly adhered to a healthy diet.

They split the group: some women walked 30 minutes a day, five times a week, while the other group of women walked 60 minutes a day, five times a week. The researchers found that all participants, whether in the 30-minute or 60-minute group, saw similar positive results. Therefore, the data suggests that when walking is combined with a healthy diet, 30-minutes a day, five times a week, may be just as good for you as walking 60-minutes a day, five times a week. By budgeting out less than three hours a week of walking, you can significantly impact your lifestyle and change your health for the better. I know everyone is busy these days, being pulled in a million directions, but I've yet to meet anyone who couldn't spare half an hour a day in order to add years of good health onto his or her life.

Do note that participants who only dieted did not see as significant of results as those that combined simple dietary changes and regular walking. That's not to say that dieting isn't important. It's simple mathematics (and I mean *very* simple, don't worry). Your body loses weight because the amount of energy (food) you put into it is less than the amount of energy you burn off during the day. If you just eat less, you'll lose some weight. If you eat the same amount as always, but exercise, then you'll lose weight. If, on the other hand, you eat less *and* exercise more, well, you can see where this is going. Again, this is why my 3-part strategy of diet, walking and resistance training is critical for maximizing results. If you want to see the best results, more quickly, then you're going to have to combine all three.

The University of Miami's study is also a classic example of why the modern "insanity" workout fads are a terrible idea for everyone. Well, a bad idea for everyone except the swindlers who take advantage of the insecurities of others, convincing people to dish out their hard-earned money for a "secret plan" that they didn't need. There's no need to spend all your free time exercising. You've got other stuff to do!

For the record, I am a bodybuilder who has to be in top shape most of the year. I carry about 5.5% body fat and weigh roughly 197 pounds. "Oh wow," you might think. "He must spend his entire life in the gym!" That's the misconception fostered by the media. I'm like you. I don't have the time to spend all day, every day in the gym just to maintain my body. Know how I do it? By working out intelligently, maximizing my results and minimizing the time wasted on exercises after I've reached my peak for the day.

I do intense resistance training about 180 minutes a week, and then I walk for another few hours a week. That's it. If you work out efficiently, that's all you need. In short, there are accountants and hockey moms working out two to three times longer than I do, and they probably don't have six-pack abs and 170 pounds of lean muscle on their frame, with the heart, knees, and lungs of a 25-year-old.

Time is not the most critical factor when it comes to exercise! Intensity under limited duration, followed by *slightly* longer bouts of moderate duration is the key. Don't worry if this is all confusing. I'll explain more later. For now, just know that the time commitment you'll need to complete my program each week is probably *much lower* than you expect. No matter how busy you are, I'm only asking for a couple of hours per week to completely reshape your body into what you've always dreamed of and to also protect your body against disease and degeneration as best as you can.

Throughout all of the studies we've discussed in this chapter, the most important factor for fat loss results, as well as long-term health benefits, is the lifestyle change. Making a healthy change doesn't have to be complicated, but it does require consistency. You have to make room in your schedule, and commit to the routine to find optimal results. Keep dieting, and stick to a plan once you've made it. Healthiness is a frame of mind, and one that gets easier to maintain the longer that you practice it. You can't just binge on healthiness—once you've made the decision, you have to be in it for the long-haul.

My three-part system addresses the lifestyle changes that you'll need to make in order to achieve all of your goals and guides you through them step by step. I can't do them for you, but I can make it as easy as possible for you to achieve your target level of fitness. Now that you understand why walking is a natural fat burner, and how walking can help your health in a dozen different ways, it's time to actually get out there and put rubber to road.

---

ii    Garcia-Aymerich, J with E Farrerro, M A Félez, J Izquierdo, R M Marrades, and J M Antó. "Risk Factors of Readmission to Hospital for a COPD Exacerbation: A Prospective Study." *Thorax* 58 (2003): 100-105.

iii    Olshansky SJ, Passaro DJ, Hershow RC, Layden J, Carnes BA, Brody J, Hayflick L, Butler RN, Allison DB, and Ludwig DS, "A Potential Decline in Life Expectancy in the United States in the 21st Century," *New England Journal of Medicine* 352:11: 1138-1145.

iv    Kriska, Andrea M., and Aramesh Saremi, Robert L. Hanson, Peter H. Bennett, Sayuko Kobes, Desmond E. Williams, and William C. Knowler. "*Physical Activity, Obesity, and the Incidence of Type 2 Diabetes in a High-Risk Population*". *American Journal of Epidemiology* 158 (2003): 669-675.

v    Diabetes Prevention Program Research Group. "Reduction in the Incidence of Type 2 Diabetes with Lifestyle Intervention or Metformin." *New England Journal of Medicine*. 2002; Vol. 346: 393-403.

vi    Dempsey, Jennifer C. with Tanya K. Sorensen, Michelle A. Williams, I-Min Lee, Raymond S. Miller, Edward E. Dashow, and David A. Luthy. "Prospective Study of Gestational Diabetes Mellitus Risk in Relation to Maternal Recreational Physical Activity before and during Pregnancy", *American Journal of Epidemiology* 159 (2004): 663-670.

vii    Nurses' Health Study. "Some Highlights." Accessed July 15, 2012. <http://www.channing.harvard.edu/nhs/?page_id=197>

viii    Speck, RM with KS Courneya, LC Mâsse, S Duval, and KH Schmitz. "An Update of Controlled Physical Activity Trials in Cancer Survivors: A Systematic Review and Meta-Analysis." *Journal of Cancer Survivorship* 5 (2011): 112.

ix    Sesso, HD with RS Paffenbarger, Jr. and IM Lee. "Physical Activity and Coronary Heart Disease in Men: The Harvard Alumni Health Study." *Circulation* 102 (2000): 975-80. Accessed at <http://www.ncbi.nlm.nih.gov/pubmed/10961960>.

x    Kagan, Abraham. *Honolulu Heart Program: An Epidemiological Study of Coronary Heart Disease and Stroke*. Taylor & Francis, 1996.

xi    Derby, Carol A. with Beth A. Mohr, Irwin Goldstein, Henry A. Feldman, Catherine B. Johannes, and John B. McKinlay. "Modifiable Risk Factors and Erectile Dysfunction: Can Lifestyle Changes Modify Risk?" *Urology* 56 (2000): 302-306.

xii    Ruffin, Richard and Paul D. Thompson. "Can Exercise Prevent the Common Cold?" *American Journal of Medicine* 119 (2006): 909.

xiii    Voss, Michelle W. with Ruchika S. Prakash, Kirk I. Erickson, Chandramallika Basak, Laura Chaddock, Jennifer S. Kim, Heloisa Alves, Susie Heo, Amanda N. Szabo, Siobhan M. White, Thomas R. Wójcicki, Emily L. Mailey, Neha Gothe, Erin A. Olson, Edward McAuley, and Arthur F. Kramer. "Plasticity of Brain networks in a Randomized Intervention Trail of Exercise Training in Older Adults." *Frontiers in Aging Neuroscience* 2 (2010).

xiv ☒ Raji, Cyrus with Kirk Ericson, Oscar Lopez, James Becker, Caterina Rosano, Anne Newman, H. Michael Gach, Paul Thomspon, April Ho, and Lewis Kuller. "Physical Activity and Gray Matter Volume in Late Adulthood: The Cardiovascular Health Cognition Study." Presented November 28, 2010 before the Radiological Society of North America, Inc.

xv Dunn, Andrea L. with Madhukar H. Trivedi, James B. Kampert, Camillia G. Clark and Heather O. Chambliss. "Exercise Treatment for Depression." *American Journal of Preventive Medicine* 28 (2005): 1-8.

xvi Peacock, Jo, Rachel Hine, and Jules Pretty. "Got the Blues, Then Find Some Greenspace." *Mind Week Report* 1.0 (2007).

xvii Mayo Foundation for Medical Education and Research. "Walking for Fitness, Taking Steps in the Right Direction." 2002.

xviii Bond Brill, J with AC Perry, L Parker, A Robinson, and K Burnett. "Dose-Response Effect of Walking Exercise on Weight Loss. How Much is Enough?" *International Journal of Obesity* 26 (2002): 1484-93.

# Chapter 3

## The Warrior's Walk

I'm hungry. It's the worst part about losing weight, but it's a reality of everyday life while I'm working through this program. I. Am. Famished. I'm more than halfway to my target weight, but recently things have seemed to slow down a bit and my body cries out for sustenance. The program still works great, yet each day seems a little bit harder. I can't give in.

This is the hump. If I can make it through the next week or two, it should be smooth sailing from there. For now, though, I know that my former weight is still just hanging out around the corner. I've gotten rid of it for the moment, but it's just waiting for me to invite it back in for dinner like an old friend. "Oh, hi Jon, fancy seeing you here. What's for dinner? Three cheeseburgers? Sounds delicious. I just thought I'd move back in to your waist area for a while, or maybe flesh out that gut again." I absolutely cannot let that happen.

I must be ever-vigilant for the time being. I'm right on the cusp of losing the weight and getting in shape entirely. It would still be all too easy to slip up now and fall right back into old habits. I've seen it happen too many times with other people I know. I don't want the weight back. I'm just getting to the point where I can walk to the store without stopping for breath, where my feet don't hurt all the time, and where getting up off the couch is easily managed. To people who are in shape, these things are taken for granted. For me, these are luxuries I refuse to give up.

Moreover, I refuse to give up on myself that easily. I've never been too good with failure, and I won't let weight loss be one of the things I've retreated from just because it got "too hard." Nothing is too hard as long as I lay my mind to it. Every day I wake up and repeat to myself, "You can do it, Jon. You can lose this weight." Every time I am tempted to eat more, the same words come to mind. Every night before I fall asleep…well, you get the picture.

I start to find hobbies to keep the hunger at bay. I do a lot more reading than I used to, especially of medical journals. I remind myself why I'm losing the weight in the first place. I write down goals for myself: long-term goals on one side of a sheet of paper, short-term goals on the other. A person without goals is a person who is destined to fail at whatever venture they choose. I make a daily celebration of striking goals off my list. Each crossed-out goal is another reminder that I'm making progress. I can and *will* beat this affliction we call obesity.

I am a weight loss machine. I am a fighter. I am a survivor. I am a warrior. I am a new man.

• • •

Losing even a small amount of weight can have a large impact on your health, both physically and mentally. Losing larger amounts of weight? Well, that's like being handed a brand new lease on life. Suddenly, everything seems a bit more possible than it did before. You have more energy, more concentration, and a more positive outlook on everything.

While there is no downside to losing weight, however, it's still an incredible lifestyle change. Hunger and exhaustion during the beginning stages of the program are going to seriously test your mettle, and perseverance will only come if you're adequately prepared beforehand. In that vein, it's important to set goals for yourself in order to keep everything on track. You don't want to reach your second week and realize that you don't know why you're really putting yourself through this.

Let's pretend for a bit that you're an athlete, and I want you to tell me about your goals. I'm guessing that they will be something similar to: when you're exercising, your goal is generally to maximize your lean muscle, increase your cardiovascular conditioning to the max, and just all-around kick butt. In other words, you want to whip your body into shape.

Those goals are mine, as well, so I can relate. The good news is, your goals are entirely attainable with a little bit of self-discipline and a lot of walking. In fact, you already *are* an athlete, of sorts.

The smart athlete wants to preserve his/her joints and tendons. This allows for a more intense involvement in your sport of passion. If you are injured, whether in the short-term or long-term, that is going to prevent you from competing. It's going to hold you back from doing the things that you love. Whether you're a professional athlete or not, the preservation of your body so that you can do more important things is always a priority. We're trying to get your body in *better* shape, not injure it. As I've already mentioned, my sport of choice is bodybuilding. For many of you reading this book, the "sport" may be weight loss.

Weight loss... *a sport?* Don't shake your head at me. I fully believe that weight loss is, indeed, a sport. Not only is it a sport, but it's one of the hardest ones you could take part in. Weight loss is one of the few activities that require mental, physical, emotional and even spiritual energy on a 24/7 basis. Even though you may have people supporting you, fundamentally you are on your own. Nobody else can lose this weight for you. Weight loss, unlike, say, basketball, is not a part-time hobby—it's a full-time bloody battle. Even tiger-tamers get the day off sometimes.

Since you have to eat, you are battling the most vicious of demons: *hunger.* If you've ever been hungry before, well, be prepared. Not only are you going to be hungry while you're losing weight, you're going to be hungry all the time. To lose weight, you have to feed your body less than it wants. It's going to want you to wake up at two in the morning, coaxing you to go eat that cheeseburger, but you can't.

You wield the sword of discipline and smart eating like Thor swings his mighty hammer, and you do it in the face of constant temptation. As I said earlier, food is everywhere these days. It's harder to escape from the constant reminders of food than it is to actually exercise. You struggle valiantly against the forces of resistance, be it iron in the gym, or rubber exercise bands in your home. It's all the same—you're asking your body to exceed its state of homeostasis by a country mile. You're pushing beyond your comfort zone, progressively and consistently. Just when you think you cannot get another repetition out, just when you think that all hope is lost and you're going to have to turn back, you force your body to give even more from the depths of god-knows-where.

Sounds like one hell of a sport to me. Don't ever sell yourself short. I know it's hard when you lack confidence, but the old "fake-it-until-you-make-it" still applies here. You're an athlete if you're using The Mighty Three—diet, resistance training, and walking—to shape your body into what your mind desires. You're a freakin' warrior. You would have made Achilles proud. The Vikings would have welcomed you gladly into Valhalla.

So, be proud. Take this task as seriously and as passionately as you should—as you must. Put that armor on and hoist your weapon. You're a fighter now, and you have to act like one.

The smart warrior guards his/her body, saving it for the time when the true battle needs to be fought. In my case, that battle is between me and a 300-some-odd-pound bar filled with iron plates. For you, it may be a battle of the kitchen condiments, the struggle of food choices, or another sport of choice. It may even just be the battle to get in and out of your bed comfortably every day. This is no laughing matter; approach each new struggle with your weight loss as if it's a battle in an ongoing war. Keep at it long enough, and you're going to win.

There will be good days and bad days (maybe even a lot of bad days). Some days it's going to be hard for you to even find a reason in exercising anymore. I'm telling you, don't get discouraged. The worst thing you can do is give up on yourself. I believe you can do this, and you should, too.

From this point on, the exercise average people call "walking" will be known as *WARRIOR WALKING*™. We need an extraordinary name for extraordinary exercises, so welcome to the Jon Benson Warrior Walking Protocol. It's going to challenge every notion you have about the benefits and capabilities of the simple and everyday task we've so far known as walking.

For me, Warrior Walking fits the weight loss battle like a Spartan's chest plate. Walking is nature's miracle exercise. It's what we were designed to do, and doing it keeps us in top shape both mentally and physically. No other exercise can give you the same benefits that walking can.

Walking provides almost exclusive fat-burning power, yet preserves precious muscle mass, protects and strengthens tendons for that next session under the weights, and even enhances my recovery so that I grow stronger instead of more weary. It rests the mind at the end of a long day. It provides a catalyst for productive company with a loved one. It quiets my thoughts first-thing in the morning. It helps me be more productive by keeping my brain alert and focused. It helps me keep up with this fast-paced world without even breaking a sweat.

As if that wasn't enough, walking helps get me ripped-up lean. Sure, the diet and resistance training remain necessary components, but I always begin with walking, and I usually end with it as well (meaning I walk in the morning and at night when getting into top condition). Walking gets the fat loss going after a layoff, and walking takes those last few pounds off right before a show or a photo session.

Walking, when approached like a warrior, will do the same for you.

# Chapter 4

## Power In Your Stride

The gym regulars all know me by now. Walking in, I'm met with "Hey Jon!" and "How's it going, Jon?" from all sides. The gym I exercise at is more like a family than your typical gym. Over the years, we've all helped each other through the rough patches that come with keeping in shape. When I've gone through slumps (it happens to everybody), their camaraderie was what kept me coming back to the gym.

I've also witnessed plenty of these guys turn into warriors themselves, and some of them have even adopted my walking exercises into their own routines. When these guys first came into the gym, they were soft and rounded from their office lifestyles, always the ones to take that extra donut or drink that mid-afternoon soda. Now? Well, now there's not much that could stop any of them. Maybe a bear, though I think for old time's sake I'd still put money on my gym buddies. They have trained their bodies to work like automatons.

Except Ron.

Ron Runalot is one of the few regulars at the gym who never seems to lose a pound. He comes into the gym at almost the same time that I do every day, pumped up and ready to go. He doesn't even bother to chat before he jumps on the treadmill, throws on some tunes, and is off to the races. Ron hits the treadmill at a blistering pace that would frighten even Usain Bolt. *Slam slam slam slam* his feet smash against the treadmill with fury. I've never felt so bad for an inanimate object before in my life. This guy, to any casual onlooker, is going to get in shape. "This is a guy who knows how to work out," you might think when you look at him.

So why hasn't Ron dropped a pound in years? He certainly throws off enough sweat (believe me, I take an unwanted shower in it every day). As I said, at a glance you might think that Ron is working harder than anyone else at the gym, but his body certainly doesn't show it. Ron goes faster than I do, goes longer than I can, and leaves the gym, bagel in-hand.

Let's not mince words here. Ron is FAT. F-A-T *fat*.

If you think I'm being harsh, I am—but only to make you chuckle, and to prove a point.

• • •

## Never Confuse Effort With Results

If you take one thing from this chapter (or even this book), this is it. Don't be fooled by appearances. The body is more complicated than people give it credit for, and it is to their detriment. You can't just pound away at a treadmill and lose weight; there's actually such a thing as working out "smart," and all it really requires is a basic understanding of how your body functions.

It seems like all that excessive exercise-training that boosts your heart rate over 65% of its maximum capacity for too long and too often, would lead to incredible weight loss. After all, you must be burning a ton of calories, right? Actually, there's a good chance that it's *preventing* you from burning fat.

Say what?

I cannot count how many times I've seen this happen. It's a mistake that many beginners make when they start exercising regularly for the first time. When your sink breaks, you ask an expert how to fix it. If your television breaks, you do the same. For exercise, though, people think that it's self-explanatory. You just move your body around, sweat a bit, and that's exercise. An expert could tell Ron what he's doing wrong and adjust his routine accordingly. Luckily, you have me to tell you so that you don't make the same mistakes as Ron.

Sure, Ron works hard, but he's working against himself. Remember what I said earlier about burning sugar versus fat? Well, Ron is putting his body squarely into a state where sugar is being consumed much more than fat. So, his body then craves...what? Sugar! Carbohydrates. Tons and tons of carbs.

If you run a lot, expect to crave carbohydrates. There's a reason that most runners eat plates of pasta before their big races. Your body loves to use them during strenuous exercise because they're a quick and easy form of energy. On the other hand, consuming high quantities of carbohydrates will make most people gain weight. In essence, Ron is training his body to get fatter by demanding him to eat more of the foods that are causing his weight problem to begin with. More bagels, more soda, more pasta, more donuts—you get the picture. Ron is probably very confused about why he isn't losing weight. He's burning calories, right? Well, yes, but from the exact wrong place. Talk about a hamster running on a wheel!

Our approach is quite different. Don't be a Ron. Remember, we're *warriors*. We're ruthlessly efficient. We do not have time to waste burning sugars just so that we can eat them again that night. That makes no sense, and isn't going to help you burn the weight that you want. We do not care what exercise looks like—we care about **results.** Plus we also want to have some of Ron's stamina and cardiovascular health in the process. We want it all... and guess what? We're going to get it. Here's how: we are going to walk, but with power and purpose.

As you may have gathered by now, this is not about a casual stroll in the park. Although that is pleasant, and often recommended for lowering stress, it will not accomplish our goal of shedding that prehistoric body fat and keeping it off for good.

No, for that we need power. As I said, we are going to walk like warriors. Think about ancient soldiers marching off to battle. Did they stop to smell the roses? No, they marched with a purpose and determination—the same determination that you need to have to lose weight.

You're going to walk with the same power that your ancestors did when they walked off to face the enemy.

It does not matter how old you are, or how in-shape you are at the moment. In fact, that information is totally irrelevant when it comes to losing weight. All you have to do is generate more calorie-burning power than the food that you're taking in. Anyone, and I mean *anyone*, has the ability to generate more power than his or her average output. For example, if we measured your average ability to generate power during a walk as a three, using a scale of 1-10, then I'm asking you to bump that slowly over time up to a five...then six...then seven...and so on.

If, on the other hand, you're already in great cardio shape, fantastic. In that case, you already understand all about needing power and determination in your exercises. Walking, when combined with a few tricks I've developed, will get the job done for you, as well. At that point, you're just trying to maintain your level of fitness instead of ramp it up. Just make sure that you're always putting in a full effort.

Our strides will be long and deep, not short and stiff-kneed. Power comes from your hindquarters, and we'll be asking a lot of that area in the coming weeks. In fact, you're going to feel sore in muscles that you never even knew existed, if you're doing this course correctly. This is a good type of sore, though. At the end of a long walking routine, you should feel as if you accomplished something that day. Those aching legs are your gold stars for the day's achievements.

Of course, we will start you off at the correct point of entry. We do not want a beginner doing 15-grade incline long-strides at 4 miles per hour, just like we don't want an accomplished athlete idly meandering up the street without a care in the world. Whatever level you're at, you're going to be sore a lot and you're going to sweat a lot. Don't worry, beginners, you'll be getting faster and stronger in leaps and bounds. Soon, you'll be hanging in there with the pros.

As you will see in the videos I've produced, assuming you decided to add them to your order, I attack the treadmill at times like it's my sworn enemy. These are the times where I let the treadmill know who's boss, and I really put my body through its paces. At other times,

I back off and let my body catch up again. This is known as *interval training*. Interval training is the secret weapon of the fat-burning stars.

Interval training mimics our friend, the caveman. Remember those tigers from earlier? Walk with brisk and powerful strides, followed by very short bursts of faster, higher-grade "walking climbs." In this way, you'll most accurately replicate the way that our bodies evolved. Interval training allows your body to run in the most efficient way possible, because thousands of years of evolution led it to this system in the first place. It's a system that shows up in all exercises, nowadays, not just walking. The benefit of walking, however, is that we still keep our bodies burning fat exclusively instead of switching to sugars.

Interval training can be done outdoors, or, more easily, on a gym-quality treadmill. While walking outdoors is great, because you can exercise from your home without any type of special equipment, more advanced walkers may find that the treadmill gives them more control over their intervals. Personally, I use a treadmill most of the time nowadays, and save outdoors walking for especially beautiful days or a special occasion. However, you're free to do either as you see fit. Luckily, the barrier of entry for walking is practically nonexistent, even if you can't afford an expensive gym membership or a personal treadmill. I'll give you routines for both, along with beginner, intermediate and advanced protocols in the next chapter. For now, I just wanted to let you know what to expect, and what to avoid.

After a Warrior Walking session, which lasts anywhere from 15 minutes to 45 minutes, you will be drenched in sweat. You can walk for longer if you'd like, but I rarely do. Remember all those studies from earlier? Time is not the most important factor here. Just make sure that you are walking with intensity.

Regardless, if you completed the day's program successfully then you will feel thermogenic waves of heat running through your body, signaling you that the fat-burning process is now in high gear. *Thermogenesis* literally means "the creation of heat." A calorie is a unit of heat, states of thermogenesis generates the fire in which calories are burned. Think of it as a nuclear furnace, right inside your own body. It might feel uncomfortable, but just remember that it's your body's way of saying, "Thanks for letting me burn all this fat." That heat means that you've won your battle for the day, and you'll eventually come to love that feeling.

You may even notice your body is in a state of euphoria or bliss after a Warrior Walking session. This sensation is colloquially known as "runner's high," although in this program you will not be running. Don't tell your body. It doesn't know the difference. Runner's high is a side effect of your body releasing endorphins into your bloodstream during and after a workout. Endorphins are responsible for pleasant feelings and also help with pain management. The runner's high phenomenon is your body's way of rewarding you for a hard day's work, sort of like a genetic Skinner box. Your body wants to get you addicted to that feeling so that you'll keep working out.

Just let it happen and enjoy those good feelings. I promise that, despite all the scary jargon, it's a good thing. You may be wondering, even this late in the book, if it would just be faster to run. Well, the answer is: yes and no. If that seems like a cop-out to you, just bear with me for a minute. I think the question is a good one, but it's a bit more complex than "one is better than the other." In fact, both exercises utilize your body in such different ways that they're hardly comparable, even though to the layman, running just seems like faster walking.

Running versus walking is, in fact, an age-old question at this point. Thousands of people have weighed in on the topic over the years, and the Internet has only made the debate even more chaotic. People appear all over the Internet purporting to have "the answer" to the question of running versus walking the same distance. Like most controversial subjects online, it can be hard to wade through all the mess and figure out what the right answer is.

It's true: running, if done correctly, can burn calories faster than walking. It makes sense, right? You're moving twice as fast, so you burn calories approximately twice as fast. Running burns calories quickly, but as I covered earlier, those calories come more from glycogen (stored sugar) instead of from stored body fat. Uh-oh. Combined with the fact that running is replete with injuries, burn-out, and can actually *reverse* the metabolic effect you're looking to achieve (long-term fat-burning), walking is probably the wiser choice.

But walking "normally" burns fewer calories. This unfortunate fact is due to the fact that your heart rate is rarely elevated, and the muscles in the upper body are less active (thus, burning fewer calories). Remember those fat golfers from earlier? A normal stroll across the green is not going to magically burn off that cheeseburger from lunch. You'll expend some energy, but not as much as you would by running. Do you feel out of breath after a leisurely walk through the park, stopping to sniff the roses whenever you'd like? Well, maybe, if you're as overweight as I used to be, but that's beside the point. Ideally, a moderately paced walk is not going to leave you out of breath, and that's a sign you aren't burning an optimum amount of calories.

So how fast do you have to walk? The President's Council on Physical Fitness and Sports found if you can achieve a one-mile brisk walk in about 15 minutes, you would burn about the same amount of calories jogging a mile in 8.5 minutes, if that helps put perspective on things. The old adage, "walking a mile or running a mile burns the same amount of calories," is not technically true—running still comes out slightly ahead.

But hold your horses—not everything is as it seems, even when we're talking about the experts. The reason is simple: they are comparing running against "normal" walking—***not* Warrior Walking.** We're not just walking like we're in a hurry, or have a purpose (descriptors often used to describe power-walking). We are walking to stalk down our prey. And, our prey is that lean, mean physique we've longed for since our self-consciousness began back in the high school locker room.

This is not just your typical early-morning power-walk around the mall in a Day-Glo tracksuit. If you are a beginner to exercise, or you're currently out of condition, don't worry—you'll be starting nice and easy. Just keep on persevering, though, and eventually your inner warrior will reveal him/herself in a wonderful way. One day, you're going to wonder (like I do) how you ever got so out of shape, or why you dealt with it for so long.

I'll put the calories burned during a Warrior Walking session against the average jogger any day of the week and twice on Sunday. This is especially true of the Advanced Warrior Walking protocols covered in the next chapter. Yet even basic Warrior Walking takes greater advantage of the lower body muscles by removing momentum from the equation. Momentum, normally a friend of ours, is actually an enemy for our weight loss goals. Momentum allows you to coast on previously exerted energy, preventing you from burning all the calories that the action would normally take. Momentum wants to help you exert less, but exercise demands that you exert more. For our fat burning purposes, we want to keep friction in the picture at all times.

Warrior Walking also peaks your heart rate high enough and for just long enough as to not waste your muscle tissue. This alone, over time, will allow you to burn far more calories during a Warrior Walk than a Joker's Jog, all while protecting yourself from the injuries (tendinitis, shin splints, and sore knees, just to name a few) that plague virtually every runner I know.

On top of that, for most people, walking is just far more enjoyable. It's no wonder that so many people quit running after just a few weeks. It's an unpleasant exercise, and one that your body was only meant to sustain for brief moments at a time. For many others, walking is the only exercise that's even doable. That was my case many years ago, so if that's your situation then fret not. Before you know it, you'll be doing whatever exercise suits your fancy.

Running is so passé. Warrior Walking is the future, baby. I suggest you enjoy it.

# Chapter 5

## The Warrior Walking Routines

Imagine, briefly, a second quiet morning, almost exactly like the one I described in the first chapter. This morning, however, takes place some months after I began walking for my health. I can hear the crashing of the ocean not far off. In my hands I carry a bottle of water and that same old portable CD player. In brand new gym clothes, I stride down the quiet suburban sidewalk. Nowadays, I walk powerfully, with a presence. These streets, which up until recently seemed like soaring mountain peaks, now reveal themselves as gentle rolling hills. Sweat drips off me, but it's the healthy sweat of a proud warrior instead of the sickly sweat of a body thrown up against the ropes.

I still have a little ways to go before I reach my target level of fitness, but my friends are already amazed at the difference. I'm easily in the best shape of my life, even if I'm not quite there yet. A few of them asked me for my "weight loss secret," but didn't believe me when I told them that I lost most of it by walking. On the other hand, I've come across a few of them walking in the mornings now. The person I was a year ago is almost unrecognizable. Unimaginable, even. The memory of being 62 pounds overweight is a bad, but distant nightmare, kind of like having a dream that you missed a test long after you've already graduated.

The same man from earlier in the year is outside watering his lawn, as he always is at this hour. His car still gleams in the driveway and his polo remains crisp. In fact, not much has changed from that beautiful June morning a few months ago except for me. I wave while I walk on by, easily cresting the peak next to his house and starting the last portion of my routine as I work my way downhill. "Beautiful day, huh?" I call out to him.

"Couldn't ask for better, I think," he responds.

That's all we have time for, as I rapidly pass his house. I can almost hear the Doppler effect when I speed by. In a year or two, at this rate, our conversations will be reduced to just a quick, "Hi."

Nowadays, I walk with a confidence and vigor unknown to me fifteen years ago. I do most of my walking on the treadmill because I like the control that it gives me over my workout, but I still occasionally choose a particularly beautiful day to do my walking outside. My body, once frail and decrepit, is still in great shape even though I'm in my late forties. In fact, my body would make the average lazy twenty-year-old jealous, even though I'm more than twice that age.

Walking has given me a new life entirely. I can't believe I wasted so much time doubting myself earlier on in life; all I needed to do was get out there and start walking. If someone had told me then what I know now…well, let's just say it wouldn't have taken me thirty-one years to get in shape. Don't let it take you that long, either.

• • •

We're heading into the final stretch now, so let me just quickly recap what we've learned so far:

1. Walking is the exercise our bodies were designed to do. Brisk walking with spurts of higher intensity exercise will cause the fat to melt off your body, leaving you with the toned and muscular physique that you've always dreamed of. All it takes is self-discipline and routine exercise.

2   Walking will do much more for your body than just burn fat. In fact, it helps you prevent or minimize effects from a variety of different diseases, including strokes, cancer and mental degradation. Walking for your health keeps every part of your body in a better position to fight illness.

3   Walk like a warrior. You are waging a war against your weight, and only determination can help you come out on top. Take up your arms and fight against hunger and exhaustion. Keep going until you think you can't anymore, and then go one step further. This program will leave you tired at first, but you will be satisfied with the result.

4   Never confuse effort with results. This is a big one. Don't think that just because Ron Runalot is out there going a million miles per minute, that you should be too. You should definitely be working hard, but you should also be working efficiently. Don't fall into habits that will actually work against you in the weight loss battle.

I only repeat this information because it's important to keep in mind for the upcoming chapter, the big one, the coup de grace: this chapter contains all the information you need to get out there and start walking on your own. That's right, you're ready now. If you've been comfortably curled up on the couch and reading this, well, it's time to get up and get in gear. I have nothing else to teach you in this book except the actual program. Within these upcoming pages is all the information I have on my "secret program," my "miracle weight loss tip."

That makes it sound like it should be hidden in some tomb somewhere for treasure hunters to find, but I assure you that my program is no secret. In fact, if you still don't know what my program consists of, you probably didn't read much of this book (or even look at the title, for that matter). It's simple; it's accessible, and still, it all boils down to one thing: walking.

Again, this is not just any walking. It's Warrior Walking. It's walking "with a twist," if you will. Nevertheless, it's fundamentally about putting one foot in front of the other at a brisk pace.

Warrior Walking is broken up into distinct intervals. Remember that interval training we talked about earlier? Well, here is where it comes into play, and it's *very* important to the program. The intervals I've specified in Warrior Walking are designed to (a) warm your body up and get it ready for exercise; (b) take advantage of the "long, brisk" walking that burns exclusively fat for fuel; and (c) provide the short-duration climbs and bursts required to kick calorie burning up to the max and give you all the heart-healthy cardiovascular benefits of intense exercise, all in a fraction of the time. Doing just one of these intervals is not going to do much for your body, but routinely doing all three is going to kick its fat-burning potential into high gear.

As I covered earlier, this chapter will detail beginner, intermediate, and advanced level Warrior Walking protocols, utilizing your choice of a gym-quality treadmill or indoor/outdoor walking. However, allow me to first demonstrate a typical Warrior Walk (WW from here on out) as I perform it. This is an intermediate WW protocol (I mix intermediate and advanced up during the week) on a treadmill, and it will give you an idea of how WW intervals are performed:

### Warrior Walk: Intermediate Treadmill Protocol

| Time | Incline | Speed | Stride |
|---|---|---|---|
| Warm-up | | | |
| 4 min | 2 - 3 | 3 - 3.3 mph | Brisk; normal (warm-up) |
| Climb Interval 1 | | | |
| 1 min | 6 | 3.6 mph | Long/push from glutes |
| Steady State Interval 1 | | | |
| 3 min | 2 - 3 | 3 - 3.3 mph | Brisk and Long |
| Climb Interval 2 | | | |
| 1 min | 5 | 3.6 mph | Long/push from glutes |
| 1 min | 10 | 3.9 mph | Very Brisk |
| Steady State Interval 2 | | | |
| 3 min | 2 - 3 | 3 - 3.3 mph | Brisk and Long |
| Climb Interval 3 | | | |
| 1 min | 10 | 3.6 mph | Long/push from glutes |
| 1 min | 15 (max) | 3.9 mph | Extremely Brisk |
| Steady State Interval 3 | | | |
| 3 min | 2 - 3 | 3 - 3.3 mph | Brisk and Long |
| Cool-down | | | |
| 2 – 5 min | 3 down to 0 | Down to 1.5 | Slow, Deep, Stretch |
| **TOTAL TIME: 20-23 minutes** | | | |

Phew, that's a lot of information in one little table. As you can see, this is not your father's walk around the block. Don't worry, though, I'm going to walk you through it all step-by-step and make sure that you understand everything before I turn you loose to walk on your own.

First of all, make sure that you always warm up before you start walking. I recommend that you start off every exercise routine with some brisk, but still relatively mild, walking, just to get your muscles and heart warmed up. We don't want to jump right in to our peak performance level without a warm-up, because that could lead to injuries.

I vary the intensity of the walk after four minutes with my first interval climb at an incline level of six on the treadmill. For this climb, I typically increase the speed by .3 miles per hour, and I recommend that you also perform a .3 mph increase no matter what speed you started at. This interval lasts for only one minute, but it's going to get your blood really pumping and increase the rate at which your body burns energy. It lasts for such a short time, however, because we want to bring the body back to a lower tier of exertion *before* it switches over to burning sugar. If we were going to put in all of this effort just to burn sugar, we might as well be running, and I don't think anyone wants that.

After the first climb, there is a lengthier period of steady state walking for maximum fat burning. This interval is three minutes long, and as you can see, takes place on a much smaller incline. Steady state walking is what you'll be doing most of the time in my program. The climbs last for a very short amount of time, with longer stretches of steady state in between. This type of walking, which combines a brisk pace with very long strokes, is where the "power" aspect of Warrior Walking comes in. Don't just walk like you're out for a stroll in the park. There will be plenty of time to do that later.

In my typical daily routine, this first section of steady state walking is followed by, not one but *two*, climbing interval bouts. The first minute of these climbs is spent at level five, and the second at level ten. My speed increases as well, to almost four miles an hour, during the level ten climb. By now, as you can imagine, I'm breathing fairly hard. When I was 62 pounds overweight, I couldn't even have handled this section of the workout, let alone the full length.

We then, of course, return to a steady state walking section. Catch your breath a little. Let your heart catch up with the rest of your body. Hopefully by the end of this section you're feeling a bit more relaxed and prepared, because the last section is going to be a tough one.

The final interval in this twenty-minute protocol is a repeat of the second, only the climbs are at levels ten and fifteen (fifteen being the highest incline this particular treadmill goes to). The speed increases yet again on the level twenty climb, back to 3.9 mph. A walk this brisk, for me, is almost a light jog in terms of speed, but the long, deep strides make this much more powerful and calorically demanding than any jog I've ever done. Remember, we want friction. If you feel yourself needing to jog or run to keep up, slow the treadmill back down a bit. It's better to keep your body burning fat at a slightly lower level than to start running and just end up burning sugar.

One last steady state section before we finish up. By now, you should be pretty exhausted. These last few minutes of steady state walking is normally the hardest part of my workout, because I am already exhausted from everything that came before and my legs and lungs are burning from the level fifteen climb. However, it is vital to complete the section in order to maximize your fat burning potential. Your body is already in a heightened state of energy-burning, thanks to those climbs we did. Now it just needs you to keep walking the weight off.

Finally, I always conclude with at least a two-minute cool-down, during which I gradually reduce the incline and the speed. Like the warm-up, this section is important to help prevent injuries. The cool-down brings your body back down to its normal state, letting your lungs and heart slowly grow accustomed to the lessened level of activity. We want your body to know that the exercise is over for now, and it can take a rest.

Do note that my steady state walking is done with a graded incline of anywhere from level two to level three. This level is based on my mood, on my energy level and on timing. If I'm performing this after an intensive weight-training session, I'll keep it around level one or two, and may even lower the speed to 3 mph, with a max of 3.3 mph on the graded climbs. Why? The reason is that my heart rate is already

## THE WARRIOR WALKING ROUTINES | 49

150 or greater from my training session. I do not want to push my body too far over the lactate threshold, or else it will start burning sugar instead, so I hold back a bit and allow my heart rate to drop.

My heart rate goal for steady state is between 125-145. I don't mind going a tad higher than the 65% MHR (Maximum Heart Rate) recommended for steady-state cardio, because, frankly, I enjoy the added challenge. Plus, I have a rather high resting heart rate, so I go by my breathing. As long as I'm able to easily carry on a conversation, I know I'm in the right steady state zone. It's easy to get caught up in the numbers, but just know that you don't have to unless you enjoy it (I kind of do).

My goal for the climbs is as high as I can get my heart rate safely. After a leg workout and then a bout of walking, I've seen my heart rate as high as 175 on the last climb. That's fairly high for a guy who is almost 49 years old, despite my conditioning and the shape that my body is in.

But why only a minute at this rate? Is this enough to get the cardiovascular benefits of, say, a half-hour jog?

Believe it or not, it **is.**

Dr. Richard Winnet is a huge proponent of the *GXP Cardio Protocol*, which is a 9-15 minute workout very similar in nature to our own Warrior Walking Protocol. Winnet wished to discover how much the average participant could raise their MET, which is a measure of oxygen consumption and cardiovascular or aerobic capacity, just by using GXP. Winnet found that subjects often improved their MET from 10 (considered average) to 12.5 (their genetic limit) in fewer than 18 months.

If your MET level increases to its genetic limit, there's simply no room for improvement anymore. It is physically impossible for your heart to get any better at that point. These participants weren't busting their bodies in the gym for hours a day, either. Dr. Winnet's subjects trained only two or three times per week, nine minutes per session, and still were able to achieve their genetic maximum in under a year and a half.

Thus, another blow to those "insanity" principles I talked about earlier—you know, busting your butt for 90 minutes a day, five days a week in front of your TV? "Insane" is an appropriate term, indeed. There is absolutely no reason for you to be working your body that hard. A much more moderate time commitment is all you need to make in order to tap the full genetic potential of your body. Again, never confuse effort with results. It's a saying that I live by, and you should too. Just because other people look like they're working harder, doesn't mean that they're working smarter.

To finish out my explanation of the Warrior Walking Protocol, let me say this: I'll do a 20-minutes post-workout Warrior Walk three days per week. I do not need more than this, unless I'm weeks out from a photo shoot or competitive event.

On my off-days, I will usually do *two* cycles of this same twenty-minute protocol. When I start over after the initial twenty minutes, I will occasionally bump the steady-state grade up one level to push my fat burning potential even higher. In other words, if I walked at level two during the first twenty minutes of Warrior Walking, I'll walk at level three for the second. On these days I'll end with a full five-minute cool down, ensuring that my heart rate drops to at least 120-130 before leaving the treadmill.

Other than those very special cases where I'm prepping for a bodybuilding event and need to be even more lean than usual (occasions which you may or may not have), I can get by and maintain my physique with only this very moderate time commitment each week.

## "Why use a treadmill?"

That's a fair question, especially since I live at the top of a bluff overlooking the Pacific Ocean in Malibu, California. You would think that would be beyond ideal for walking, and you'd be correct. The weather is awesome, and the beauty is staggering.

However, my goal when I'm walking nowadays is not to look at nature's beauty and be inspired. My goal is to walk like a Warrior—

efficient, ruthless, and measured. I want to know exactly how hard my body is working at all times.

Do not let my preference deter you from walking outside, however. You most certainly *can* walk like a Warrior outside. If you're on a trail with natural hills and valleys, for example, you'll out-Warrior me any day. I just enjoy pushing the buttons, having control over the graded inclines, and measuring my heart rate. Plus, the gym is merely a block away, and I have a lot of friends there to help inspire my workouts. Having a friend there to support you can be a huge help when you're trying to burn off the pounds or eke out that last minute of exercise. I recommend that whether you're working out at the gym, at home, or outside that you find someone else who is like-minded about getting in shape so that you can motivate each other. It will be a huge help in the long run.

## The Warrior Workout Walking Routines

On the pages that follow, I'll be covering all the protocols for beginners, intermediate-level exercisers, and advanced athletes. You'll note that, although I prefer a gym setting and a treadmill for ultimate control, outdoor protocols are also included.

Be sure to gently stretch and get your feet and calves nice and warm before you start. Since my walking is done post-weight training, this is not a concern for me. However, if you begin cold, please consider a 5-minute stretching session prior to your Warrior Walk. As I discussed earlier, failure to warm up can result in injuries, scuttling your weight loss endeavor. Always err on the side of caution when it comes to exercise. We want to protect our bodies—after all, they're the only ones we've got.

Finally, please note this important fact: you do not have to do every interval if your body tells you to stop, or if you're just having a bad day. We all have them, and they're nothing to be ashamed of. Pushing your body to the limit is a great feeling, and even necessary sometimes for our weight loss purposes. However, we want to always be sure that we're not pushing beyond the limit. Ten minutes of exercise is better than nothing, and usually you'll come back stronger than ever. Stop and rest if you feel nauseous or dizzy. Listen to your body! It's better to be safe and take a break for the day than it is to be sorry and end up in the hospital with a bunch of concerned faces looking down at you.

## Warrior Walk: Beginner Outdoors Protocol

NOTE: You will want to walk on a slight incline. Pick a street, sidewalk, or trail that has a slight incline. Also, we will be measuring speed with simple terms like "slow" or "brisk." Slow=low to moderate breathing. Medium=moderate breathing. Brisk=moderate to semi-heavy breathing.

| Time | Incline | Speed | Stride |
|---|---|---|---|
| Warm-up | | | |
| 4min | Slight | Slow | Normal |
| Speed Interval 1 | | | |
| 1 min | Slight | Medium | Long/push from glutes |
| Steady State Interval 1 | | | |
| 3 min | Slight | Slow | Normal/push from glutes |
| Speed Interval 2 | | | |
| 1 min | Slight | Medium | Long/push from glutes |
| 1 min | Slight | Brisk | Normal stride |
| Steady State Interval 2 | | | |
| 3 min | Slight | Medium | Brisk and Long |
| Cool-down | | | |
| 2-5 min | Walk downhill | Slow | Slow, Deep, Stretch |
| **TOTAL TIME: 15-20 minutes** | | | |

## Warrior Walk: Beginner Treadmill Protocol

| Time | Incline | Speed | Stride |
|---|---|---|---|
| Warm-up | | | |
| 4min | 0 | 2-2.5 mph | Normal/brisk (warm-up) |
| Climb Interval 1 | | | |
| 1 min | 3 | 3mph | Long/push from glutes |
| Steady State Interval 1 | | | |
| 3 min | 1 | 2.5mph | Brisk and Long |
| Climb Interval 2 | | | |
| 1 min | 4 | 3-3.3mph | Long/push from glutes |
| Steady State Interval 2 | | | |
| 3 min | 1 | 2.5mph | Brisk and Long |
| Cool-down | | | |
| 2-5 min | 1 down to 0 | Down to 1.5 | Slow, Deep, Stretch |
| **TOTAL TIME: 15-20 minutes** | | | |

## Warrior Walk: Intermediate Outdoors Protocol

NOTE: You will want to walk on a slight incline. Pick a street, sidewalk, or trail that has a moderate incline. Also, we will be measuring speed with simple terms like "slow" or "brisk." Slow=low to moderate breathing. Medium=moderate breathing. Brisk=moderate to semi-heavy breathing.

| Time | Incline | Speed | Stride |
|---|---|---|---|
| Warm-up | | | |
| 4min | Moderate | Slow | Normal |
| Speed Interval 1 | | | |
| 1 min | Moderate | Medium | Long/push from glutes |
| Steady State Interval 1 | | | |
| 3 min | Moderate | Slow | Normal/push from glutes |
| Speed Interval 2 | | | |
| 1 min | Moderate | Medium | Long/push from glutes |
| 1 min | Moderate | Brisk | Long/push from glutes |
| Steady State Interval 2 | | | |
| 3 min | Moderate | Medium | Brisk and Long |
| Speed Interval 3 | | | |
| 1 min | Moderate | Medium | Long/push from glutes |
| 1 min | Moderate | Brisk | Normal Stride |
| Steady State Interval 3 | | | |
| 3 min | Moderate | Medium | Brisk and Long |
| Cool-down | | | |
| 2-5 min | Walk downhill | Slow | Slow, Deep, Stretch |
| **TOTAL TIME: 20-23 minutes** | | | |

## Warrior Walk: Intermediate Treadmill Protocol

| Time | Incline | Speed | Stride |
|---|---|---|---|
| Warm-up | | | |
| 4min | 2 - 3 | 3-3.3 mph | Brisk; normal (warm-up) |
| Climb Interval 1 | | | |
| 1 min | 6 | 3.6 mph | Long/push from glutes |
| Steady State Interval 1 | | | |
| 3 min | 2–3 | 3-3.3 mph | Brisk and Long |
| Climb Interval 2 | | | |
| 1 min | 5 | 3.6 mph | Long/push from glutes |
| 1 min | 10 | 3.9 mph | Very Brisk |
| Steady State Interval 2 | | | |
| 3 min | 2–3 | 3-3.3 mph | Brisk and Long |
| Climb Interval 3 | | | |
| 1 min | 10 | 3.6 mph | Long/push from glutes |
| 1 min | 15 (max) | 3.9 mph | Extremely Brisk |
| Steady State Interval 3 | | | |
| 3 min | 2–3 | 3-3.3 mph | Brisk and Long |
| Cool-down | | | |
| 2-5 min | 3 down to 0 | Down to 1.5 | Slow, Deep, Stretch |
| **TOTAL TIME: 20-23 minutes** | | | |

## Warrior Walk: Advanced Outdoors Protocol

NOTE: You will want to walk on a slight incline. Pick a street, sidewalk, or trail that has a steep incline. Also, we will be measuring speed with simple terms like "slow" or "brisk." Slow=low to moderate breathing. Medium=moderate breathing. Brisk=moderate to semi-heavy breathing.

| Time | Incline | Speed | Stride |
|---|---|---|---|
| Warm-up | | | |
| 4 min | Steep | Medium | Normal |
| Speed Interval 1 | | | |
| 1 min | Steep | Brisk | Long/push from glutes |
| Steady State Interval 1 | | | |
| 3 min | Steep | Medium | Normal/push from glutes |
| Speed Interval 2 | | | |
| 1 min | Steep | Brisk | Long/push from glutes |
| 1 min | Steep | Very Brisk | Normal Stride |
| Steady State Interval 2 | | | |
| 3 min | Steep | Medium | Brisk and Long |
| Speed Interval 3 | | | |
| 1 min | Steep | Medium | Long/push from glutes |
| 1 min | Steep | Brisk | Normal Stride |
| Steady State Interval 3 | | | |
| 3-5 min | Steep | Medium | Brisk and Long |
| Speed Interval 4 | | | |
| 3-5 min | Steep | Very Brisk | Long/push from glutes |
| Cool-down | | | |
| 5-10 min | Walk downhill | Slow | Slow, Deep, Stretch |
| **TOTAL TIME: 28-38 minutes**  (Repeat 2x if super-advanced) | | | |

## Warrior Walk: Advanced Treadmill Protocol

| Time | Incline | Speed | Stride |
|---|---|---|---|
| Warm-up | | | |
| 4min | 4 | 3-3.3 mph | Brisk; normal (warm-up) |
| Climb Interval 1 | | | |
| 1 min | 8 | 4 mph | Long/push from glutes |
| Steady State Interval 1 | | | |
| 3 min | 4-6 | 3.6 mph | Brisk and Long |
| Climb Interval 2 | | | |
| 1 min | 8 | 4 mph | Long/push from glutes |
| 1 min | 12 | 4.3 mph | Very Brisk |
| Steady State Interval 2 | | | |
| 3 min | 4-6 | 3.6 mph | Brisk and Long |
| Climb Interval 3 | | | |
| 2 min | 15 | 4-4.3 mph | Long/push from glutes |
| Steady State Interval 3 | | | |
| 3 min | 4-6 | 3.6 mph | Brisk and Long |
| Climb Interval 4 | | | |
| 1 min | 15 | 4.5 mph | Long/push from glutes |
| Steady State Interval 4 | | | |
| 3 min | 4-6 | 3.6 mph | Brisk and Long |
| Cool-down | | | |
| 2-5 min | 4 down to 0 | Down to 1.5 | Slow, Deep, Stretch |
| **TOTAL TIME: 24-27 minutes** | (Repeat 2x if super-advanced) | | |

# Chapter 6

## Conclusion

It's time for your first walk. After years of doubt and self-consciousness, you're ready to get out there and prove everyone wrong. Sure, it's going to be a long and hard process, but you have all the confidence in the world that you'll be successful. You have your husband/wife/parents/children on board as support in this difficult time; you've picked out a beautiful walk for this morning or you have your treadmill all set up, and you've learned all that I can teach you.

Pull on a t-shirt or tank top and some gym shorts. Know that, soon, these will be too large, and you'll have to purchase some new ones. Next, lace up your best, most comfortable shoes. Before too long, the soles will be worn through and falling apart from all the miles put on them.

You straighten up and look in the mirror, trying to imagine what you're going to look like in a few months. Looking back at you is a complete stranger. Wait, not a complete stranger. It's you, but in the best shape of your life. Instead of gym clothes, the mirror shows you decked out in a warrior's armor, head topped with a plumed, golden helmet.

When you put your headphones in, suitably bombastic music from your favorite epic film blares out (bonus points if it's something like

*Spartacus* or *Gladiator*). The person in the mirror raises a spear-clenched hand, saluting you and your valiant efforts.

• • •

It sounds silly, but the above story is what you're going to need to think of in order to get through the next couple of months and reach your weight loss goals. If I've said it once, I've said it a hundred times, this program necessitates an entire lifestyle change. You're not battling foes from a distant land. You're battling your body. If anything, that's even harder to accomplish. Your body is going to scream out for attention. It will try to beg and plead for mercy. It will remind you of how good you used to feel when you ate terribly and didn't exercise.

Don't listen.

The body is the trickiest foe imaginable. It will do whatever it can to get what it wants, and you will need to be constantly vigilant in order to prevent relapses. Walking is only half the battle. The other half is developing the self-determination and discipline to ignore your body when it cries out for more food or says that you'll never get in shape. You can and will get in shape, if you follow my program. I went from 62 pounds overweight to a body that anyone would be jealous of. If I can do it, you most definitely can. Lose that extra paunch, throw nature's knapsack out the window, and get your body whipped into the shape that it's capable of. Drag it, kicking and screaming, into the best shape it's ever been in.

With that in mind, I cannot stress this point enough: *walk like a Warrior, look like a champion.* If you walk like a mall shopper, you'll look like a mall shopper. If you walk like a fat golfer, you'll look like a fat golfer. Even if you're 90 and frail, walk within your abilities, but walk with *power*. Walk with total intention. Walk like you cannot wait to get wherever you're going. Walk like you own the joint. Walk like you just conquered the world. Walk like you just defeated your greatest foe. No matter what your age, weight, gender, ethnicity, or level of fitness, you are a Warrior now, and weight loss is your arena.

## CONCLUSION | 61

To be a complete Warrior, you'll need to take a serious look at your diet and resistance training. I promise, you can do this. It may sound daunting if you're just starting out, but trust me: it will soon be one of the high points of your day. Pick up my other two books. They're just as charmingly written as this one is, and will make both diet and resistance training easy and interesting to follow. My goal here is to inspire you to get your body as in shape as mine is.

Take a look at my picture:

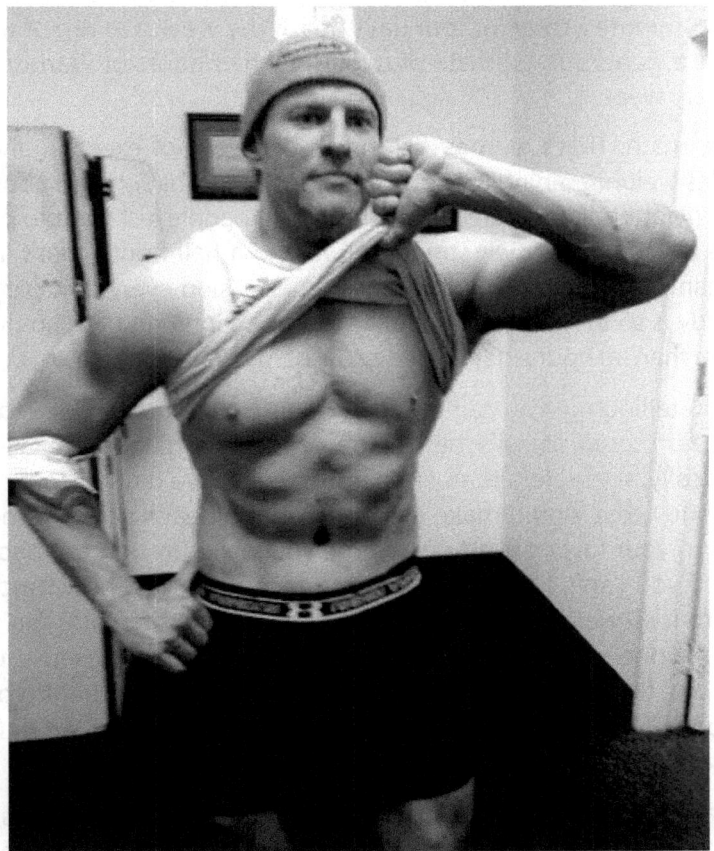

I'm just trying to show you what this program has accomplished for my own body and what it could accomplish for yours. This picture was not taken either before or for a contest. I didn't prepare for it in any

Get Your 3 FREE Bonus Fat Burning Training Videos: www.VelocityHousePresents.com/BensonAmazonBonus

special way, didn't bring in some expert to do special lighting and make my muscles pop out more, didn't pay some computer whiz to manipulate my body in Photo Shop. There was no gluing of my head on some other guy's body. In fact, I'd say that this particular picture could not be more "low-rent" if I were watching *Jersey Shore* in the background. I just think it will help prove my point.

You have to realize that I'm in the gym about 120 minutes *per week*, not counting Warrior Walking. Due to my schedule, I'll often combine workouts (I have more free time in the gym since this is my job) and train 45 minutes, three or four days out of the week. On top of that, I'll include a generous estimate of two and a half hours of Warrior Walking every week.

Do the math: That's **at most** 5.5 hours per week of exercise, and that includes weight training for bodybuilding. You probably need about half of the weight training that I do; after all, most people just want to bulk up a little and build up their strength. Five and a half hours, that's literally less than the average American watches television every day, per week. My body is so in shape that I use it in competitions, and I still only work out less than an hour a day, including all of my Warrior Walking.

Are you telling me you can't spare a measly 45 minutes a day to get a body that could literally be on the cover of a magazine? Or, more realistically, spend less than 30 minutes a day, five days per week, and get a body that would make everyone on the beach green with envy, and turn your lover's head every time you walk through the bedroom door? If you can't, I think you need to reconsider just how much you want to lose weight. I've said it before and I'll say it again: I've yet to meet anyone whose life is so busy that they have an excuse to not work out that moderate amount every week. You'll thank yourself later on in life, when your body is still in good health instead of falling apart at the seams.

You can do this. All you need is a plan. Just go get the blueprints you'll need for all three phases if you don't have them already. This book for walking, and the others for your diet and resistance workouts:

# Now

Go take what's rightfully yours
the body you've always wanted
and enjoy the spoils of victory.

**Here's to your inner Warrior!**

www.ingramcontent.com/pod-product-compliance
Lightning Source LLC
Chambersburg PA
CBHW071412040426
42444CB00009B/2210